KETO FOR WOMEN OVER 50

THE COMPLETE KETOGENIC DIET COOKBOOK TO PREVENT DIABETES, LOW CARBS, AND TO HAVE A HEALTHY LIFESTYLE. INCLUDING A 28 DAY MEAL PLAN AND 34 DELICIOUS RECIPES.

Gena Long

Copyright © 2020 by Gena Long. All rights reserved. No part of this book may be reproduced or transmitted in any form or by any means, electronic or mechanical, including photocopying, recording or by information storage and retrieval system, without the written permission of the author.

Editing by Gena Long

Table of Contents

INTRODUCTION 5

WHAT'S THE KETOGENIC DIET? (THE KETO DIET) 11

BENEFITS OF KETO 19

HOW KETO BRINGS WEIGHT LOSS 31

THE YES OR NO OF KETO FOODS 35

FOODS TO ENJOY ON THE KETOGENIC DIET 37

FOODS ON THE MODERATION LIST 44

FOODS TO AVOID 47

WHAT TO LOOK OUT FOR IN SOME KETO FOODS 51

RECIPES 61

28 DAYS PLAN 131

INTRODUCTION

Did you ever want more energy in your day and feel better and look better? Many people have come up with a simple diet to achieve a better life. Sounds unrealistic, I know. However, it is conceivable to acquire energy, feel better, and look better and change your eating habits. There's no magic pill. Rather it's as simple as developing an eating plan that gives the nutrients your body needs.

What's that magic plan of eating? It is called the Ketogenic Diet. This eating method is not so new and has existed for thousands of years. Modern society, unfortunately, selects convenience foods that are generally loaded with carbohydrates and refined sugars.

Eating is often done on the run today. Convenience is what sells, and the producers satisfy the demands of the consumers. These convenience foods come with preservatives, coloring, adding refined sugar, salt, and grain processing. Though our schedule may be convenient, these foods are not convenient for our bodies to process.

The Ketogenic diet may sound complicated and technical; however, very literally, this diet feeds your body's foods that can be processed easier. The human body is made to function using fuel food, which, in effect, gives us energy. The Ketogenic Diet optimizes that process.

A ton of readers may not think about the ketogenic diet. This chapter talks about some broad thoughts on ketogenic slims down and characterizes terms that may be valuable. In the broadest terms, a ketogenic diet is an eating routine that makes the liver produce ketone bodies, moving the body's digestion away from glucose and towards the heavy use.

In particular, a ketogenic diet limits sugar under a specific level (normally 100 grams for each day) and instigates a progression of alterations. Protein and fat intake differ, as indicated by the calorie counter's objective.

Be that as it may, a definitive determinant of whether an eating regimen is ketogenic is the nearness (or absence) of starches. The body runs under 'ordinary' dietary conditions on a blend of starches, protein, and fat. When starches are expelled from the eating regimen, the little stores in the body quickly become exhausted.

The body is, in this way, compelled to locate an alternative fuel to give energy. One such fuel is free fatty acids (FFA), which can be found in most body tissues. Not all organs can utilize FFA, however. The mind and sensory system, for instance, can not utilize FFA for fuel; in any case, ketone bodies can be utilized.

The ketone bodies are a result of the fragmented liver corruption of FFA. They fill in as fat-inferred, non-starch fuel for tissues, for example, the cerebrum. At the point when ketone bodies are shaped at quick levels, they aggregate in the circulation system, which triggers the creation of a metabolic state called Ketosis. Simultaneously, the utilization and creation of glucose are diminishing. The breakdown of protein to be utilized for vitality alluded to as 'protein saving' is diminishing. With an end goal to lessen muscle to fat ratio while staying away from loss of fit weight, numerous people are pulled in to ketogenic eats less.

The alterations referenced above are activated primarily by ketogenic slims, affecting the degrees of two hormones: insulin and glucagon. Insulin is a storage hormone that moves supplements out of the circulation system into target tissues. For instance, insulin makes glucose be put away as glycogen in the muscle, and FFA put away as triglycerides in the fat tissue.

Glucagon is a fuel-preparing hormone that invigorates the body to separate the put-away glycogen to give glucose to the body, especially in the liver. As the eating regimen takes out starches, insulin levels lessening, and glucagon levels rise. This caused an expanded arrival of FFA from fat cells and expanded consuming of FFA in the liver.

What inevitably adds to the advancement of ketone bodies and Ketosis's metabolic state is the fast consuming of FFA in the liver. Some different hormones are likewise influenced, notwithstanding insulin and glucagon, all of which assist move with filling utilize away from sugars and toward fat.

The body has four fuel sources: carbohydrates, fat, protein, and ketones. But what exactly are ketones? Ketones develop as fat is broken down inside the body. The effect of a Ketogenic diet is that fat and ketones are the body 's principal source of power. Consuming more fats, some protein, and minimal carbohydrates are the secret to following a Ketogenic diet. In this way, the body can be in a state of nutritional Ketosis.

You need to explore the benefits/risks with your doctor before you start any diets. It's essential to consider the effect a diet can have on your body and your health. This will help you pick a safe diet and deliver optimum results. Eating a ketogenic diet is not simply eating a diet low in carbohydrates. Consider not counting carbohydrates but being aware of your body and responding to the foods you eat. Do you just give yourself the nutrients you need?

A ketogenic diet is a lifestyle change and a change of mindset. The blood sugar levels can drop rapidly when the body uses carbohydrates to convert glucose to energy. The signs are sugar and starch hunger and cravings.

Drops in blood sugar are minimized on a ketogenic diet. This is because fats and ketones are used as fuel rather than as quick carbohydrates to burn. Foods that cause cravings for sugar, salt, and fats hinder weight loss. These addictive foods trigger food over-consumption, which never gives a true sense of satisfaction. Most often, the culprits are processed foods.

These foods can be avoided on a ketogenic diet, and so are the resulting cravings and hunger for junk food. Instead of calorie counting, adhere to foods that are found in nature and are easy to pronounce. Inflammation is caused by foods such as grains, dairy, and refined sugar. Inflammation hinders weight loss and causes your body to build up toxins. The toxins will be removed after the Ketogenic Diet starts, and inflammation will decrease.

Whether you're taking the first steps of your New Year's resolution or just looking to modify your food intake and get healthy, the Ketogenic Diet is a great choice for you.

Throughout this book, you'll be exposed to some of the most easily prepared mouth-watering recipes, and before you know it, the Ketogenic Diet will cease to be a diet; it will become a way of life.

As you will find, a Ketogenic regiment is about high fat, low sugars, and a sound measure of protein, permitting your body to depend on fats as vitality instead of consuming the starches. Also, the additional time you spend on the program, you'll feel progressively solid.

However, the important thing is when you begin the Ketogenic Diet. It's the consistency that is something to remember. Of course, when the opportunity presents itself, you can find it difficult not to indulge in the occasional cheat meal, for instance during the holidays or on an outing with friends. While your body should be able to bounce back fully once you return to the diet, you must adhere to it as strictly as possible to sustain a high metabolic rate.

WHAT'S THE KETOGENIC DIET? (THE KETO DIET)

Despite many different types of diets you've undoubtedly heard of in your life, there's bound to be a few new to you. One of these may be the Ketogenic Diet, otherwise called the Keto Diet, a low-sugar high-fat routine.

The ketogenic diet is not a new-cached fad diet based on shaky nutritional science. Since ancient times, it has been around using the diet as part of holistic epilepsy treatment for ancient Greeks. Indeed, over here in the states, in the 1920s, it was a standard method of treatment for childhood epileptic seizures.

Unfortunately, with its penchant for immediate effects, this natural way of therapy had to give ideas to pharmaceutical science's modern advances. Thankfully, the ketogenic diet again made its way back into the mainstream, and possibly for very good reasons! The basis of the diet is basically to activate the mechanisms of the body's fat-burning to feel what the body needs for energy all day. That means the fat you eat and the fat stored in your body have all become fuel stores that your body can tap on!

The theory behind the high-fat, low-carbohydrate ratio is that the body relies on fat for energy rather than carbohydrates. Therefore the body becomes leaner as a result of less fat being stored in the body. In a perfect world, the Keto diet ought to permit the body to go into Ketosis, or a metabolic state where ketones are expended, which are fats. Many who follow the Keto diet often eat just the right amount of protein the body needs every day.

Unlike some of the other diets that exist, the Keto Diet doesn't focus on calorie counting. Instead, the focus is on the food's fat, carbohydrate, protein makeup, and the weight of the food.

A traditional Ketogenic diet meal will have a high-fat, low-carbohydrate ratio. It could include a healthy protein serving such as chicken, some fruit or a vegetable rich in protein, and a high-fat portion that could be butter. The high-fat portion of this diet typically comes from the food-making ingredients; this may include heavy cream, butter, or buttermilk and creamy dressings like ranch.

Why go for the Ketogenic Diet?

Scientists have found, over the years, that picking the Ketogenic Diet has numerous advantages. The primary hypothesis was that the eating routine would cause the development of cholesterol in the body, in this manner prompting coronary illness because of the high-fat substance of the nourishments that individuals on a careful nutritional plan could devour.

As an ever-increasing number of specialists investigated the eating regimen, they found that there are inborn points of interest to this sort of diet, in any case. For a certain something, the body can utilize fat for vitality rather than sugars.

Therefore, because there is such a modest quantity entering the body, the body doesn't rely upon carbohydrates. Henceforth, it would have the option to store ketones-the fats-for later vitality utilization. Another advantage is the way that the body won't be as eager, and subsequently, individuals on the Keto diet are at a lower danger of eating off their regiment.

Since the Keto diet supports the utilization of various nourishments wealthy in proteins that work to control hunger, the body enters the condition of ketosis-basic among the individuals who quickly normally and along these lines don't require a lot of food to prop it up. What better than being on a solid eating regimen and not having steady aches of craving?

At last, critical is the medical advantages gave by the Keto Diet. Individuals who follow the Keto diet dispense with boring sugars, for example, bread and pasta, totally and supplant them with non-dull vegetables like broccoli, asparagus, carrots, etc. Such vegetables are stuffed with nutrients and supplements that help a solid body and are additionally much lower in calories.

Just as helping victims, the Keto diet is likewise suggested for cancer patients from infections, for example, epilepsy. As work has appeared, cancer cells thrive in parts of the body where there's a lot of glucose, which is the thing that structures starches. Should the body devour less, subsequently, sugars will be less glucose, and cancer cells won't have the option to create and endure a while later.

Little wonder that this diet helps you with weight loss even for those stubborn, hard to lose fatty areas. That may be one reason you chose this book and looked into embarking on the ketogenic path, or you may have learned stuff from your social circle about how the keto diet normalizes blood sugar levels and optimizes your cholesterol readings, and you're fascinated.

How about stories of type 2 diabetes being reversed just after this diet alone and stories of some cancers being stopped or tumors shrinking because of the positive effects of a keto diet? And we must not ignore the associated reduction of the risk of cardiovascular disease due to diet!

All of the benefits mentioned above stem largely from a single substantial ketogenic diet cycle. The game's name is Ketosis. Ketosis is a condition in which the body produces molecules called ketones that are created through the liver. It is designed to give the cells and organs energy and substitute glucose as an alternative fuel source. We get most of our energy from glucose in our traditional, carbohydrate-rich diet, converted from the carbs we eat during meals.

Glucose is a rapid source of energy where insulin is required as a kind of messenger that tells the cells to open up and allow glucose to flow in such a way that it can be used as a fuel for the mitochondria, otherwise known as the cells' energy factory.

The more carbs we ingest, the greater the amount of glucose in our blood, which means that the pancreas needs to produce more insulin to facilitate energy production from the available blood sugars. In a corps in which the metabolic function is still normal, the cells readily accept the insulin produced from the pancreas, leading to the efficient use of blood sugar as energy.

Our cells can become desensitized with insulin, leading to a situation where the pancreas is forced to pump more and more insulin into the body just to clear and normalize the blood sugar levels. Insulin de-sensitivity or insulin resistance is generated primarily because of

Continuous increased blood glucose presence, usually caused by carb-rich food ingestion. Think of the cells in your body as a bouncer at a club, where you have to enter the club and pay a fee. Here you play the role of glucose, and insulin is the fee required for joining the club. If your club frequency is in line with the standard, the bouncer does not notice anything odd and will not increase the entry fee.

However, if you show up just about every night clamoring to be left in, the bouncer knows your desperate need and jacks up the insulin fee correspondingly to let the glucose in. The entry fee gradually becomes higher and higher until the insulin source, which is the pancreas, no longer produces any. This is where the situation is diagnosed as type 2 diabetes, and the usual solution would involve a lifespan of the medicines or a shot of insulin.

The crux of the matter here lies in the body system's presence of glucose. Our blood sugar levels are elevated, and insulin is activated for conversion into energy and the preservation of the unused excess into fat cells any time we take in a carb-rich meal, which is not difficult in this day and age of fast food and sugar treatments. It is here where the normal furor occurs, with condemnations coming in for both glucose and insulin as the root of many illnesses and dreaded weight gain. I would like to take this opportunity to point out that insulin and glucose are certainly not the roots of all evil, as some books have made it.

To point our current diet to be the leading cause of obesity and metabolic diseases plaguing the better part of the developed world would be far more accurate—cue the ketogenic diet, which allows us to see the change for the better.

The keto diet is a diet based on fat, with a focus on being deliberately low carb. This approach is designed to reduce our intake of sugary and starchy foods that are available so conveniently. Just a fun fact: in the olden days' sugar was used as a preservative, and it's no coincidence that many of the processed foods we see today contain high levels of sugar only because it requires a longer shelf life. Foods high in sugar have also been shown to activate the brain's hedonic appetite response, effectively causing you to consume instead of actual desire for pleasure.

Studies have shown that sugar treatments are associated with brain areas that are also responsible for gambling and drug addiction. Now you know why you can't seem to stop those candied sweets popping into your mouth! So we're cutting back on the sugars, which is where fats come in to offset the body's energy needs.

On the regular ketogenic diet, 75% of your daily calories should be taken as fats, about 20% as proteins, and the remaining 5% as carbs. We do this because we want fats to become our main source of fuel, as you remember.

It is only with the combination of cutting down carbs and increasing our fat intake that we will trigger Ketosis in the body. It's either a diet that allows long-term and sustainable use, or we're starving on Ketosis. Yes, you heard me right. Ketosis is the body's natural function, which builds a buffer when food is scarce against those lean times.

BENEFITS OF KETO

A ketogenic diet isn't something that has been designed as of late. Individuals have been taking ketogenic counts calories for about 3,000,000 years, during which time our minds have been rising and developing. Presently the human mind isn't just contracting. However, cerebrum decay has become the standard as we age. We are tormented by sicknesses like Alzheimer's dementia and Parkinson 's malady.

Our brain, organs, and tissues work much better when utilizing ketones as a wellspring of fuel. The mind and the heart follow up on ketones in any event 25 percent more successfully than glucose. Ketones are the ideal fuel for our bodies, in contrast to glucose, which is destructive, less steady, additionally energizing, and abbreviates your life expectancy.

There's something called glycation, where the protein binds glucose. This cycle produces free radicals and inflammation, which are Alzheimer's markers. It's pretty easy to do a test and see if your body has this happening.

If your Hemoglobin A1c is high, free radicals increase by fifty-fold. Studies say this is a precursor to the development of brain atrophy.

Ketones are our bodies ' fuel, yet they are extraordinary for our minds too. They give substrates that help with fixing harmed neurons and layers. That is why I'm pushing a high-fat, low-carb diet for customers who have Alzheimer's (occasionally called type 3 diabetes) and seizures.

Ketones are non-glycating, which implies they have no caramelizing impact on your body. Mitochondria are our cells' energy-producing "powerhouse" factories. They work significantly better on a ketogenic diet because energy levels can increase consistently, long-lasting, and efficient. A ketogenic diet also increases our mitochondria's energetic output because of these incredible "powerhouse."

The output is increased, and an inflammatory by-product load is reduced. Glucose should be prepared in the cell first before it very well may be moved to the mitochondria plant "powerhouse."

Fat energy sources don't need this processing: for energy, they go straight into the mitochondria. Creating energy out of glucose is more intricate than out of fat, which causes you to get more energy per fat molecule than glucose. I see such a large number of clients with fibromyalgia, constant exhaustion, rheumatoid joint pain, cancer, different sclerosis, and other energy misfortune immune system sicknesses.

The ketogenic diet acts simultaneously on numerous levels, something no drug has been able to do without adverse side effects. You likely skim bored out of your mind over this information. I did the same in my biology class, certainly, when I was in high school. But this science isn't just simple. It can be quite fascinating.

Keto-adjusted eating regimens don't starve your brain and don't cause you to feel tired from the start when you're not yet to change. Give it time, and you'll have more energy than you ever imagined possible.

Risk of coronary artery disease decrease

Inflammation is the most significant contributor to risk from heart disease. A well-developed diet that is keto-adapted causes very little inflammation. Sugar and carbohydrates are the main culprits in growing the inflammation. Coronary artery disease occurs when an artery wall contains a low-density lipoprotein particle (LDL) embedded in a lesion (caused by inflammation). This particle then releases its cholesterol into the wall of the artery, which begins plaque formation.

Add fresh garlic and onions daily to the food to increase sulfur in your diet. Beware, however: cooking onions destroys sulfates for even ten minutes. Also, bear in mind that you need ample quantities of sunlight to absorb sulfur. Let us have a look! Well formulated diets which are keto-adapted:

1. Decrease muscle to fat ratio significantly more than low-fat weight control plans, in this way, reassuring the low-carb gatherings to eat until full.

2. Reduce blood sugar, and boost diabetes symptoms.

3. Increase (the right kind of) HDL cholesterol much more than low-fat diets.

4. Change LDL cholesterol pattern (the bad type) from small, dense LDL to big LDL (the very poor kind).

5. Trigger the blood pressure to drop more.

6. Lower Triglycerides in the blood.

In conclusion, well-formulated keto-adapted diets enhance all health biomarkers much more than the low-fat eating regimens despite everything suggested by specialists.

A Keto-Adapted Diet Stops Cancer Cells Feeding

A very much figured ketogenic diet has serious and fast cancer. All cells in your body, even cancer cells, are fuelled by glucose. On the other hand, cancer cells have a tremendous human defect: they don't have the metabolic versatility to be fuelled by ketones. However, they can flourish with ketones in your sound cells.

Subsequently, since malignancy cells need glucose to flourish, and starches in your body transform into glucose, cut out of sugars, disease cells kick the bucket.

Like a high-carb diet, a ketogenic diet doesn't harm our safe framework and has less free extreme harm in our cells. Free radicals are exceptionally receptive mitochondrial particles that harm the protein tissues and cell films. As we do work out, free radicals are produced.

Ketones, on the other hand, are "clean-burning fuel." If ketones are the wellspring of fuel, then the amount of ROS (number of fuel) is the same.

The oxygen-free radicals) are decreased drastically. Concentrated exercise on a high-carb diet overpowers cancer prevention agent resistances and cell layers, clarifying why extraordinary competitors have hindered insusceptible frameworks and diminished the soundness of the digestive organs.

A well-designed ketogenic diet battles these free radicals, which causes signs of aging and reduces intestinal inflammation and improves immune systems as never before.

Raising healthy fats is the healthiest way to stop feeding cancer cells.

Those who want to reduce carbohydrates in their diets are making the mistake of growing their protein take-in. Too much protein will increase glucose production via gluconeogenesis. I know I've written that many times, but people make such a common mistake when carbohydrates are cut out. Limit protein only to organic and pastured high-quality sources. I recommend 0.5 grams of protein per pound of a slender body in cancer patients averaging about 50 grams of protein per day.

Low-carb Diets ExcludeFood Groups That Are Essential

You must exclude all food products from your diet if you wish to become keto-adapted. In the main, these are starches, grains, legumes, sweets, sucrose condiments, drinks, and other high-carb foods are included. Most people with damaged metabolisms also need to get rid of fruit.

Despite the propaganda of ads for all these foods, there is no clear dietary need for them. Many of these foods were not available to humans in the evolutionary period. We have also not started consuming grains until around 10,000 years ago, and we have not started eating refined fast foods until very recently.

Sugar was a very expensive product, and cost ten times as much as milk. There's no vitamin or mineral in carb-laden products that we can't get out of meat, herbs, and vegetables in larger quantities. The diet involves no real need for foods such as grains.

Also, the grain is often considered anti-nutrient, which means it interferes with our bodies' ability to absorb nutrition. For example, grains are very high in phytic acid, a substance that hampers the absorption of dietary iron, zinc, and calcium from the diet.

Another advantage of avoiding wheat (including whole wheat) is that it can lead to improved levels of vitamin D. This is because wheat fiber intake has been shown to minimize this very significant vitamin's blood levels, low-carb diets do not include wheat and are low in phytic acid; thus, they do not produce substances that "steal" nutrients from the body.

Have you ever noticed that from Halloween until Valentine's Day, children become sick a lot? Do you blame the cold weather on that? Then again, guess. Between that time, some holidays focus on sweets. Sugar is depressing your immune system. White blood cells need vitamin C so they can protect themselves against viruses and bacteria. White blood cells require fifty times higher vitamin C concentrations inside the cell than outside, so your kids must get enough vitamin C.

At this time, he came up with his theory that high doses of vitamin C are needed to fight the common cold. We know that glucose and vitamin C have identical chemical structures, but when the sugar levels go up, what happens? Glucose and vitamin C are competing for entry into the cells.

What is more, the thing that mediates glucose entry into the cells is the same thing that mediates vitamin C entry into the cells. If more glucose is present around, less vitamin C is allowed into the cell. And not much glucose is needed either: a blood sugar value of 120 reduces the phagocytic index by 75%. Thus your immune system slows down to a crawl when you eat sugar.

Simple sugars often worsen asthma, cause mood swings; magnify personality; increase mental illness; increase fuel efficiency, nervous disorders; diabetes, and heart disease increase; gallstones grow; hypertension accelerates, and arthritis magnifies. Since sugar is deficient in minerals and vitamins, it draws on the body's micro-nutrient stores to be metabolized into the system. A cereal dish, and skim milk? A type of pop-tart? Try feeding them organic eggs with lots of omega-3 and healthy protein or my own to keep your kids healthy and focused.

Recipe for Shamrock Shake. A balanced fat and protein-filled breakfast have been shown to improve both adults' and children's concentration and achievement.

Many raw, unprocessed foods high in fat, such as eggs, meat, fish, and nuts, are incredibly nutritious and are especially rich in fat-soluble vitamins that lack low-fat diets. Not a single one of the well-formulated keto-adapted diet studies show any signs of a deficiency in nutrients.

The decrease in undesired menopause side effects

If you're a woman in your twenties, you might read this section and wonder why you'd ever want your period to come back on earth. For many other desired processes that come with it, our menstrual cycle produces hormones that create a snowball effect. Menopausal women often suffer from dry tissue and reduced libido (not to mention their body temperatures going through the roof and sometimes gaining weight in the belly).

Many of my clients complain during menopause that they lose some of their feminine features on their face and body and are taking on a more masculine look. This is because their bodies mimic the production of masculine hormones (less healthy progesterone and estrogen). And those undesired effects are only external effects.

Within, there are also some serious problems, such as bone loss, decreased collagen and elastin production, and reduced muscle mass. A woman's mental and emotional well-being can be shattered by the unpredictable hormonal highs and lows and clothing that doesn't fit the way it used to. The fact that menopausal women have low estrogen has been grossly simplified; owing to this simplification, these women are often given estrogen as a hormone replacement that can cause further estrogen dominance.

For menopausal women, the first hormonal adjustment is degradation to progesterone. Not is estrogen. The estrogen levels get too high in some cases. We need to counterbalance estrogen and progesterone. When the progesterone levels drop, the levels of estrogen shoot up to compensate for estrogen maintaining dominance.

Control of convulsions, autism, epilepsy and Alzheimer's

A well-formulated keto-adapted diet has numerous benefits for neurological conditions: it relieves neuronal hunger from cognitive hypoglycemia. It stimulates the essential immune response against intracellular pathogens and helps cure infections in the brain. It does away with excess glutamate. It has been shown that feeding the ketone beta-hydroxybutyrate instead of glucose allows less glutamate to develop.

This is significant since excessive glutamate in the brain is "excitotoxic" and destroys neurons. Glutamate excitotoxicity destroys a variety of conditions including stroke, traumatic brain injury, spinal cord injury and central nervous system (CNS) neurodegenerative diseases such as Alzheimer's disease, multiple sclerosis, amyotrophic lateral sclerosis (ALS), Parkinson's disease, withdrawal of alcohol or alcohol and Huntington's disease.

Epilepsy, schizophrenia, anxiety, and other mood disorders benefit from a keto-adapted diet because it reduces glutamates' excitotoxicity.

Following a ketogenic diet can benefit from weight loss, increased cognitive performance, balanced blood sugar, and improved cardiovascular health.

Mental focus — The brain uses ketone bodies as its primary source of food, instead of glucose, on a ketogenic diet. This switch can foster more nerve growth factors and synaptic connections between brain cells, resulting in increased mental alertness, sharper focus, and enhanced cognitive abilities.

Blood sugar management — Low carbohydrate diets have been shown to help support insulin metabolism in the body. This is because the absence of dietary carbohydrates helps your body keep blood glucose levels by breaking down fats and proteins.

Weight loss — A reduced ketogenic calorie diet promotes body fat as fuel, and clinical studies support its use for weight management. A ketogenic diet may also help to suppress the appetite and reduce cravings.

Increased energy — Carbohydrates only go so far throughout the day to sustain energy, and especially during a workout. In Ketosis, instead of glucose, your body uses fat as a fuel to provide the brain with a consistent supply of the ketone bodies necessary to sustain physical performance.

Cardiovascular and metabolic health — A ketogenic diet has been shown to help promote lipids' metabolism in the blood and fatty acids.

HOW KETO BRINGS WEIGHT LOSS

One of the first things we always lose when we embark on a ketogenic diet is water weight. Glucose is stored as adipose fats by the body, but a small supply of glucose is stored as glycogen, which consists mostly of water. Glycogen is meant to deliver rapid bursting energy, the kind we need when we are sprinting or lifting weights.

As we cut carbs, the body turns to glycogen as the first pool of energy supply, so the initial stages of water weight are lost. For many, this initial burst of lost weight can be a morale booster, and it's a good sign of what's going to happen to people who stick to the keto diet. Water weight easily gets lost on a side note and gained. This means that for folks who initially see some results on the keto diet and then decide to get off the bandwagon, the chances are their weight would balloon back up once carbs become the daily caloric mainstay.

What happens next for those who adhere to the ketogenic diet is the fat burning process of the body responsible for the impressive weight loss results seen by many. In this adipose, the basic premise is still the same.

The fats are now regulated by the body's organs and cells as energy sources, resulting in a normal state of fat loss and, subsequently, weight reduction.

Fat burning isn't the only reason a keto diet displays weight loss. Suppression of hunger and increase of satiety after meals are also reasons why people are better able to lose weight when feeding. One of the central tenets of weight loss has always been the adage of eating less and doing more. The whole idea is to create a calorie deficit so that the body needs to rely on its stored energy supplies to make up for the expenditure required.

That sounds easy and simple on paper, but it could be as difficult as scaling Mount Everest for anyone who has been through situations where you had to curb your eating on a hungry stomach consciously!

With the ketogenic diet, you know that you will have normal hunger suppression because of the hormone change that regulates feelings of hunger and fullness. Also, the food we usually eat while on a diet helps with weight loss. It is known that fats and protein are more satiating and fulfilling than sugary carbs.

When we switch to a high-fat diet while cutting down on the carbs, at the same time, we achieve two things pretty much. Restoring carbs, especially sugar stuff, reduces the eating impulse because you feel like it, not because you're starving. Jacking up the intake of fat also creates a much faster satiety effect, and makes you feel full. That's why many keto dieters say they can go on two and a half or even two meals a day without feeling the slightest pinch of starvation.

We account for a daily calorie intake ranging from 1,800 to 2,000 calories on our keto meal plan, and we don't use calorie restriction to minimize weight. The reality is that those tiny and innocent-looking snacks that occupy the time between meals will not feature much in your life when you're experiencing fullness and satisfaction from your meals! Think about it: donuts, cookies, and cakes, which are the usual go-to treats, get cut out only, so you're less likely to give in to hedonistic hunger caused mainly by the same sugar treatments! That goes a long way in cutting excess calories that would otherwise have turned into adipose fat.

To sum up, the ketogenic diet makes meals without the usual calorie limitation of other foods contributing to weight loss. It also offers a helping hand in producing results on hunger suppression, so you don't have to deal with those dastardly hunger pangs! There is also the issue of carb cravings that could theoretically ruin any diet. This helps us to experience natural weight loss, with as little disturbance as possible to our everyday lives.

There is no need to deploy calorie counters, no need for troubled six to eight meals a day, and definitely no weird or funny exercise routines required. When you couple that with the fulfilling keto high-fat meals, you get to a situation where hunger might become a stranger.

We are getting to relearn what true starvation is like also comes off as another positive spin. We get instances of hunger on a carb-rich diet because our blood sugar levels tend to fluctuate wildly as our cells gradually become insulin desensitized. Also, sugar increases the tendency to eat on impulse, which can derail any diet! When we cut down on carbs and ramp up on the fats, we'd have to sit up and notice when we feel any hunger pangs, because those would be the right signals your body needs to refuel.

THE YES OR NO OF KETO FOODS

Let's get to the meat of things now! This chapter will begin by fleshing out the foods you'll get to know intimately. Oh yes, it will feature fatty meats and dairy products, and don't forget your fruits and greens! There's going to be another section about what kind of foods to cut down to limit your carb consumption.

The lists are intended to act as a kind of easy prim for keto-friendly foods, making it easier for you to select and identify which foods are good to go during meal times.

The normal requirements for ketogenic diet macronutrients are 75% Fats, 20% Protein, and 5% Carbohydrates.

If we translate this into a daily intake of 2,000 calories, we are looking at 1,500 calories from fats, 400 protein calories, and the remaining 100 carbs calories. With each gram of protein and carb yielding 4 calories, and each gram of fat yielding 9 calories, the whole breakdown above would end up with approximately 166 grams of fat, 100 grams of protein and 25 grams of carbs per day.

These numbers of macronutrients should be at the forefront of your mind when you begin the ketogenic diet first. Remember, always try to hit your fat requirement, limit your intake of carb, and think about how much protein you get into your system.

If your experience is anything like mine, you'll find eating enough fat tends to be a problem, at least in the initial stages. This is partly because the liquid forms contain a lot of the fat that you take in. Think of olive and coconut oils, or butter and lard when heated on the skillet, they're all high fat essential in the keto diet, but they can easily be overlooked because they're never going to be the main food. I noticed that keeping my daily fat numbers counted enabled my fat intake to increase.

On the days where the fat count is a little low, 99 percent dark chocolate and bulletproof coffee will nudge those numbers back to where they should be. Of course, many other high-fat foods can do the trick too, so let's look at them!

FOODS TO ENJOY ON THE KETOGENIC DIET

Various types of food fall within this list. Such food concepts undoubtedly advocate for high-fat content while simultaneously packaging other nutrients and balanced vitamins for use by the body.

Meats And Animal Products-Focus on grass-fed or pasture-raised fatty cuts of meat and wild-caught seafood, avoiding farmed animal meat and processed meat as much as possible. And don't forget about meats made from the organ!

- Beef

- Chicken

- Eggs

- Goat

- Lamb

- Pork

- Rabbit
- Turkey
- Venison
- Shellfish
- Salmon
- Mackerel
- Tuna
- Halibut
- Cod
- Gelatin
- Organ meats

Good Fats – Monounsaturated and polyunsaturated fats are the best fats to eat on the ketogenic diet, but there are plenty of good saturated fats. Avoid trans fats, at the risk of sounding like a broken recorder. Perhaps "avoid" is not a fitting word. It might be better to run away. Runaway from trans fats like a plague you should. Enough to say.

- Butter
- Chicken fat

- Coconut oil
- Duck fat
- Ghee
- Lard
- Tallow
- MCT oil
- Avocado oil
- Macadamia oil
- Extra virgin olive oil
- Coconut butter
- Coconut milk
- Palm shortening

Vegetables – Fresh vegetables are nutrient-rich and low in calories, making them a great addition to the diet. However, you need to be careful about carbs with the ketogenic diet, so stick to the leafy greens and low-glycemic veggies rather than root vegetables and other starchy veggies. I've put avocados in this section because some might recognize it as a vegetable even if it's a fruit.

- Artichokes

- Asparagus
- Avocado
- Bell peppers
- Broccoli
- Cabbage
- Cauliflower• Cucumber
- Celery
- Kohlrabi
- Lettuce
- Okra or ladies' fingers
- Radishes
- Seaweed
- Spinach
- Tomatoes
- Watercress
- Zucchini

Dairy Products – You can include full-fat, unpasteurized, and raw food products in your diet to handle the food. Bear in mind that certain brands will contain a lot of sugar that could increase the carb content, so look out for nutrition labels and limit your intake. If possible, go for the full-fat varieties because they are less likely to substitute the fat with sugar.

- Kefir
- Cottage cheese
- Cream cheese
- Cheddar cheese
- Brie cheese
- Mozzarella cheese
- Swiss cheese
- Sour cream
- Full-fat yogurt
- Heavy cream

Herbs and spices – Fresh herbs and dried spices are a great way to taste your food without adding significant calories or carbohydrates.

- Basil
- Black pepper

- Cayenne
- Cardamom
- Chili powder
- Cilantro
- Cinnamon
- Cumin
- Curry powder
- Garam masala
- Ginger
- Garlic
- Nutmeg
- Oregano
- Onion
- Paprika
- Parsley
- Rosemary
- Sea salt
- Sage

- Thyme

- Turmeric

- White pepper

Beverages – On the ketogenic diet, you should avoid all sweetened drinks, but there are certain drinks that you can still have to add a little more variety to your choice of liquids besides good old water.

- Almond milk unsweetened

- Bone broth• Cashew milk unsweetened

- Coconut milk

- Club soda

- Coffee

- Herbal tea

- Mineral water

- Seltzer water

- Tea

FOODS ON THE MODERATION LIST

These food items are included here as they appear to have a higher carb count. Therefore moderation is essential. However, they are full of other nutrients, and some of them throw in the extra bit of fat to help with your regular intake of calories!

Fruit-New fruit is an excellent food source. They are sadly often filled with sugar, which means that they are rich in carbohydrates. You can enjoy a few low to moderate-carb fruits in smaller amounts, but you have to watch how much you eat them!

Often, stopping them going into our mouths is very easy. "Candy of Nature" is an accurate moniker to them. With the right levels of intake, we can still get their benefits and sustain Ketosis.

Most of the fruits described below are all right for you to have a cup or so, maybe a single slice or two daily, especially when you're starting first and looking to keep your carb count low. As you advance and get better handling of your carb threshold, it's okay to increase the quantity of these foods while remaining within your carb limit package.

- Apricot
- Blackberries
- Blueberries
- Cantaloupe
- Cherries
- Cranberries• Grapefruit
- Honeydew
- Kiwi
- Lemon
- Lime
- Peaches
- Raspberries
- Strawberries

Nuts And Seeds – While nuts and seeds contain carbohydrates. They are rich in healthy fats as well. The following nuts and seeds are low to moderate in carb content, so you can enjoy them while watching your portion sizes.

Typically an ounce or a handful of nuts would be a good indicator of how much you can consume and still live in Ketosis every day.

- Almonds
- Cashews
- Chia seeds
- Hazelnuts
- Macadamia nuts
- Pecans
- Pine nuts
- Pistachios
- Psyllium
- Pumpkin seeds
- Sesame seeds
- Sunflower seeds
- Walnuts
- Nut butter

FOODS TO AVOID

There are several big categories to consider when it comes to foods that you can avoid on the ketogenic diet. First and foremost, as they are the highest in carbohydrates, you should avoid the grains and grain-based ingredients as much as possible. Choose healthy fats over hydrogenated oils, and try to limit starchy vegetables and high-glycemic fruit intake.

Refined sugars such as white sugar and brown sugar are completely restricted to sweeteners, and you should avoid artificial sweeteners.

Natural sweeteners like honey, pure maple syrup, and agave aren't necessarily bad for you, but carbohydrates are very high. Powdered erythritol, stevia, and monk fruit sweetener are the best sweeteners to use on ketogenic diets.

Stevia is a herb also called a sugar leaf. This sweetener comes in several forms, and you need to make sure that there is no artificial sweetener in whatever type you buy.

Liquid stevia extract is usually the best option, although powdered stevia extract can also be found here. Another option is powdered erythritol, which is extracted from corn, and it's usually the best way to use baked goods in recipes. As far as sauces and condiments are concerned, you must read the food label to see if the item is keto-friendly or not because brands differ significantly.

Basic condiments such as yellow mustard, mayonnaise, horseradish, hot sauce, Worcestershire sauce, vinegar, and oils are keto-friendly, in general, when it comes to such things as ketchup, BBQ sauce and salad dressings you need to be mindful of the sugar content in them.

Here's a short rundown of some of the big foods you'll need to avoid on the ketogenic diet.

- All-purpose flour
- Baking mix
- Wheat flour
- Pastry flour
- Cake flour
- Cereal
- Pasta

- Rice

- Corn• Baked goods

- Corn syrup

- Snack bars

- Quinoa

- Buckwheat

- Barley

- Couscous

- Oats

- Muesli

- Margarine

- Canola oil

- Hydrogenated oils

- Bananas

- Mangos

- Pineapple

- Potatoes

- Sweet potatoes

- Candy
- Milk chocolate
- Ice cream
- Sports drinks
- Juice cocktail
- Soda
- Beer
- Milk
- Low-fat dairy
- White sugar
- Brown sugar • Maple syrup
- Honey
- Agave

WHAT TO LOOK OUT FOR IN SOME KETO FOODS

I figured it would be fitting to share some tips and ideas on what to look for when selecting the most common and popular keto foods to prepare our meals.

Salmon – When it comes to keto-friendly food, this fatty fish has always ranked high for me. You may know it is packed with beneficial polyunsaturated omega-3 fats that boost brain health and help reduce inflammation, but it also has loads of other nutrients that the body needs.

When it comes to salmon, potassium and selenium are found in abundance. Potassium is an integral part of proper blood pressure regulation and water retention for the body. Selenium helps to maintain good bone health and also to ensure an optimal immune system.

Also, salmon contains healthy levels of vitamins B. These vitamins are crucial to energy-processing adequate food, as well as maintaining the proper function of both the body's

DNA and nervous system. Astaxanthin is present in salmon, an antioxidant that gives salmon flesh its reddish-pink hue to top it off.

This powerful antioxidant helps the health of the heart and brain and may also benefit the skin. The first thing you should take note of is the smell, to get a good quality deal.

For that matter, fresh salmon, or any fish, will not have a smell. You may smell an ocean tinge, but the fresh fish definitely won't smell fishy. You know when it's fishy that the fish isn't for you.

Next, watch out for the eyes. Look for the ones with shiny and clear eyes. Think of a film star who's torn up-those are the kind of eyes that best reveal what you're looking for. Never go for eyes that are sunken or dry. Cloudy-looking ones also make a no-go when it comes to selecting fresh fish.

Fins and gills are also areas we want to watch out for. Fresh fish have wet and whole-looking fins, which are not torn and ragged. Their gills are bright red and clean, slimy, and not brownish-grey. Finally, if you are permitted to do so, try to press the flesh and see if it bounces back like your own. Depressed and staying depressed flesh should not end up in your kitchen.

The best you can do for filet cuts is to pay attention to the color and the look of the piece. It should be vibrant and bright in color. Varied hues ranging from red to coral to pink are appropriate but note that the flesh's brightness is important. Next would be spotting any breaks or cracks in the flesh themselves.

These are signs the filet has been holding for some time and is not as new anymore. Also, any pooling of water should trigger alarm bells, because it means the structure of the flesh has begun to break down, and it's time to move on to another piece. Every 100 grams of pork belly has about 50 grams of fat in it.

You can be sure that this is a good food item to boost your daily fat count by packaging another 9 grams of protein and absolutely no carbs. On top of that, preparing delicious meals with it can be completely easy.

You should look at the color of the cut when selecting a pork belly. Go to dark red for the cuts, which are reddish-purple. Meat that is lighter in color usually means that the freshness might have faded. Greying or discoloration would certainly mean that rot has already settled in, and the meat should not be collected.

The other thing you want to look for in the pork belly is the streaky white stripes of fat present. The more streaks it usually has, the better the marbling will be, and that's good news for you. Always make sure the marbling is white because any yellow or grayish coloring would represent meat that probably has passed its date of sale.

Avocado oil – I have to be frank here and admit that this oil has been a later stage addition for me compared to olive and coconut oil. Olive oil extra virgin and flexible coconut oil have their rightful place in the staple keto food pantheon, but avocado oil might give them a run for their money.

For one avocado oil is mainly monounsaturated fat. This particular quirk ties into something really important. Like vegetable oil and even extra virgin olive oil, the oil is considered even more robust than any of its polyunsaturated fat relatives. Besides that, avocado oil is known to have a higher smoke point than most vegetable oils, somewhere around 500 degrees Fahrenheit.

This makes it a valuable addition to the kitchen since the oil has a higher heat-degeneration resistance. Add to the fact that it packs a good punch in vitamins, minerals, phytochemicals, and antioxidants. You'll know this is one oil you can use for several different applications.

Some people use it for hair and skin care, where it is known that vitamin E rich oil can easily be absorbed without additional chemicals or other potentially harmful additives. It is also a great way to boost monounsaturated fat intake with minimal inconvenience by adding oil into salads, vegetables, or fruits.

You might even want to try to drink it raw, although it doesn't work for me as I found it to be a bit too rough. Mixing it with a little lime or garlic was always what I prefer.

Now let's talk a bit about how to choose the avocado oil. Second, we want to look at the source or origin of the oil, which usually means that we need to learn where and how to grow the avocados.

In this respect, to know that the avocados were produced without any synthetic pesticides, you have to look for a certified organic mark. This means that the avocado-derived oil does not contain any substances which could affect your health.

Next, we have to look at how to remove the crude. Mechanical and chemical methods of extraction usually involve increased heat and potent chemicals to force the oil out of the mashed avocado pulp. The downside of this is that heat and chemicals can reduce the nutrients and vitamins that are beneficial in the oil. Cold pressing, known as the least damaging process out there, ensures color, smell, and taste are similar to the original seed. You get better quality oil, and you'll also enjoy more nutrients.

The last item to look at is how, or not. The oil is refined. Earnestly, cold-pressed oil, which is unrefined and obtained from certified organic avocados, would rank among the top, if not the top, levels for best results. The downside is that it has a short shelf life, and the oil smells very ... avocado-ish.

If you use it often and consider the health benefits and convenience it brings, that shouldn't be a problem. The next best thing would be to have the oil refined naturally, where typically the manufacturers do straining and filtering to extend the shelf life. Remember always that the more refined the oil, the less nutrition it will provide.

Always opt for oils in dark-colored glass bottles or tins before I forget. This is very similar to extra virgin olive oil, wherein the presence of heat and light. There is still a small percentage of polyunsaturated fats for avocado oil, although the majority of fats present consist of the monounsaturated variety. Therefore, it is better to err on the cautionary side and go for dark colors glass bottles.

Ghee – Since the Ayurvedic times, this substance has been near and has consistently been recorded as the mode of cooking. Ghee is clarified butter, meaning heated butter that is free from lactose and other solids in the milk. That also results in a higher point of smoke compared to butter. It can go as high as 480 degrees Fahrenheit, which means that without the possibility of oxidation producing dangerous free radicals, you can really fry or roast deeply.

Removal of lactose is excellent news for those who are intolerant to lactose, but who want to take part in the nutty and rich butter taste. Ghee can be an excellent alternative, and the taste maybe even more flavourful. Packed with multiple fat-soluble vitamins, it also contains short-chain fatty acids that enhance cardiovascular health and help fight inflammation. Ghee also has a distinct advantage that he will last about three to four weeks.

At room temperature and refrigerated, it will last for up to six months. Ghee can be found in most grocery stores, of course. Check it out in the oil area, though some places may have it in the portion of the dairy. You can always aim to get grass-fed varieties first, as with butter, to increase the intake of nutrients and reduce the chance of combining possible contaminants or chemicals. I typically go for ghee packed in tins or glass bottles for me. Lard-Lard is pig fat. Once vilified along with all the other sources of saturated fat food, lard enjoys a well-justified comeback!

Every 100 grams of lard gives you around 30 grams of immersed fat, with 10 grams of polyunsaturated fat and around 40 grams of monounsaturated assortment. No, there is nothing wrong with that. You read it right. Lard does have more monounsaturated fat than saturated fat. No big surprise why individuals from prior ages depended on fat and utilized it for all intents and purposes for most cooking and preparing stuff.

Now that we modern folk are once again coming round to lard, it was one of the richest vitamin D foods sources. You don't need to get all your vitamin D out of the sun or fish. Lard is a delicious alternative too!

Due to its higher smoke point, which stands around 375 degrees, Fahrenheit lard is also good for high heat cooking. Due to the presence of saturated fat content, which gives lard that extra layer of fat stability, there is even less chance of rancidity or free radical production. Did I already note that lard always tastes great? That's a point worth repeating, as there's just something about animal fat that gives food a really rich, flavourful texture.

Unfortunately, lard being sold in supermarkets and most stores aren't very good because they probably suffered some sort of hydrogenation to prolong shelf life. Extending the shelf life of supermarket lard comes at our own expense if we choose to add it to our meals. You really should look to your butcher or meat grocer for high-quality lard.

Good lard, also known as leaf lard, is derived from visceral fat surrounding the pig's kidneys and distant area. If that's running out, you can go for the next best alternative, which is slightly more solid lard, derived from between the back and the muscle's skin. Still refrigerate untreated or unrefined fat to preserve its freshness.

Bell peppers – These colorful vegetables add to our everyday meals in color and a crunchy taste, but they also deliver a balanced nutrient punch. Rich in vitamins A and C, and supplying us with folate and vitamin K for added good measure, bell peppers help boost our immune system and maintain healthy tissue. The antioxidant lycopene, a type of carotenoid that gives its color to the peppers, is also responsible for reducing inflammation and being an active scavenger for free radicals in the body. It is also extremely flexible, being ideally suited for the raw or lightly grilled operation. More Great News? The carb count for 100 grams of bell peppers is at a measly 5 grams, 2 grams of which consist of dietary fiber. We 're going to touch more on this dietary fiber topic and how it affects the carb count, but for now, just know that bell peppers have an intensely low carb count for all the nutritious goodness they 're packing.

The trick of selecting a bell pepper you 'd like to have on your dinner table is easy-really. Go for those with vivid, bright colors. Those with lighter colors could indicate that they are not yet ripe. Anyone with bruises and discoloration should be put aside and replaced by those with a glossy shine. Squeeze the vegetable gently to feel for skin tightness.

Another thing to note is that a ripe bell pepper feels heavier than it looks like. This is because it did not suffer from overmaturity associated moisture loss. Bell peppers can be stored for up to 10 days in the refrigerator, so be sure to pop them in the chill box once you bring them back from your grocery run.

The above list is intended to give some help regarding the physical selection of the mentioned foods. I'm sure you 'd like to keep quality and fresh food in your kitchen, and I hope this section has gone some distance to help you do that consistently.

RECIPES

Frotted Keto

Strawberry Ice Cream

This simple ice cream to make from berry is paleo-friendly, dairy-free, gluten-free, and low carb. It comes out of the blender straight out fine. Rising serving is filled with 48 percent of your daily requirement for vitamin C.

Serves: 10

Makes: 5 cups

Serving Size: 1/2 cup

Prep. Time: 5 minutes, plus 1-2 hours freezing if desired

Cook Time: 0 minutes Nutritional Facts Serving Size: 125 g Calories: 191

Total Fat: 18.4 g; Saturated Fat: 16.2 g; Trans Fat: 0.0 g Cholesterol: 0 mg; Sodium: 12 mg;

Potassium: 271 mg Total Carbohydrates: 11.3 g; Dietary Fiber: 4.4 g; Sugar: 4.8 g Protein: 2 g

Vitamin A: 0 %; Vitamin C: 48 %, Calcium: 2 %; Iron: 8 %

Ingredients:

- 2 can of coconut milk (13.5 ounces)
- 16 ounces of frozen strawberries,
- 1.5 Tablespoon stevia liquid

Optional:

- 1/2 cup fresh, chopped strawberries,

Guidelines:

1. Combine all the ingredients into a blender. Heat the mixture until smooth.

2. Put the mixture inside the ice cream maker. The process according to instructions from the manufacturer.

3. When using fresh strawberries, add these before incorporating the ice cream.

4. Serve immediately or place it in the freezer to harden for 1-2 hours.

Chocolate Ice Cream

This isn't typical of your ice cream. This recipe is dairy-free, and just 3 ingredients are needed! The use of coconut milk makes this recipe very creamy too. This one is also low carb with protein and fiber.

Serves: 4

Prep. Time: 5 minutes, plus 1 hour freezing

Cook Time: 0 minutes Nutritional Facts Serving Size: 105g Calories: 241

Total Fat: 24.7 g; Saturated Fat: 21.8 g; Trans Fat: 0.0 g Cholesterol: 0 mg; Sodium: 55 mg;

Potassium: 310mg Total Carbohydrates: 7.4 g; Dietary Fiber: 3.3 g; Sugar: 3.5 g Protein: 2.9 g

Vitamin A: 1 %; Vitamin C: 0 %, Calcium: 7 %; Iron: 10 %

Vitamin A: 0 %; Vitamin C: 5 %, Calcium: 2 %; Iron: 11 %

Ingredients:

- 2 tablespoons of unsweetened powdered cocoa
- 1 Could be coconut milk
- 1 teaspoon stevia in chocolate
- Season with salt

Optional:

- Chocolate nibs

Guidelines:

1. Mix the ingredients in a blender.

2. Pour the mixture carefully into an ice cream machine.

3. To make the ice cream follow the manufacturer's instructions.

4. Serve straight away.

Poppy Seed Lemon Ice Cream

If you're a fan of lemon poppy seed muffins, this dairy-free, a vegan cold treat will love you. Poppy seeds are very high in Calcium and Manganese. They're also an excellent source of magnesium, zinc, phosphorus, and copper.

Serves: 8–10

Prep. Time: 20 minutes, plus 1 hour freezing

Cook Time: 0 minutes Nutritional Facts Serving Size: 94g Calories: 246

Total Fat: 23.5 g; Saturated Fat: 18.6 g; Trans Fat: 0.0 g Cholesterol: 13 mg; Sodium: 24 mg;

Potassium: 219 mg

Total Carbohydrates: 4.8 g; Dietary Fiber: 1.9 g; Sugar: 2.9 g Protein: 7.1 g

Vitamin A: 3 %; Vitamin C: 10 %, Calcium: 5 %; Iron: 8 %

Ingredients:

- Three cups of coconut milk

- Seeds with 1/4 cup of chia

- 1/3 teaspoon lemon juice

- 1/2 cup honey (or 1/4 cup stevia powder xylitol or 1/4 teaspoon)

- 1/4 Ghee Cup

- 3 lbs. of poppy seeds

Guidelines:

1. Put all the ingredients in a high-velocity blender—mix for about 1 minute on high power or until all seeds are pulverized. Chill out and follow your ice cream maker 's instructions. If you aren't using an ice cream maker:

1. Freeze the blend into a rectangular container. Dump the ice cream to a clean surface when frozen, then cut it into chunks. Put the chunks in a blender for high speed. Mix, tamp down the chunks to keep the chunks in motion.

2. Pour the ice cream mixture back into the container. Again, refrigerate.

3. Alternatively, freeze, whisk and stir every 30 minutes until frozen, after pouring the mixture into a container.

Remarks:

1. If you want a smooth texture of your ice cream, add the poppy seeds. Otherwise, add them to a crunchy whole poppy seed texture right at the very end.

2. If you don't have a high-speed blender, first grind the poppy chia seeds (for a smooth texture). Pour the blender into the coconut milk, ground chia, and poppy seeds. Enable yourself to sit for a few minutes while the other ingredients are prepared.

Coconut Cream Raspberry Swirl Popsicles

Who dislikes popsicles? The ultimate snack on those warm summer days is these Keto friendly treats.

Serves: 12

Prep. Time: 20 minutes, plus 1 hour freezing

Cook Time: 0 minutes Nutritional Facts Serving Size: 73 g Calories: 89

Total Fat: 8 g; Saturated Fat: 7 g; Trans Fat: 0.0 g Cholesterol: 0 mg; Sodium: 6 mg;

Potassium: 123 mg Total Carbohydrates: 6.2 g; Dietary Fiber: 3 g; Sugar: 2.2 g Protein: 1 g

Vitamin A: 0 %; Vitamin C: 12 %, Calcium: 1 %; Iron: 4 %

Ingredients:

- 1 can of coconut milk (14 ounces) full-fat, refrigerated overnight
- 3/4 cubic teaspoon stevia
- 1/2 teaspoon extract from coconut
- 10 ounces of frozen hazelnuts

- Cup 3/4 of water

Guidelines:

1. Turn the coconut milk can chilled upside down. Off, pour the coconut water into a container, reserving it for different use.

2. Scoop out the cream of the coconut and move to a medium dish. Connect 3/4 teaspoon stevia liquid and coconut extract. Beat until soft peaks hold in the mixture. If the coconut cream is too thick to beat, add 1 tablespoon or more of the coconut water reserved to thin it up.

3. Combine the berries with the remaining sweetener and the water in a blender or food processor. Puree straight to smooth.

4. Add the coconut cream mixture into the berry mixture. Swirl the mixtures together but don't thoroughly blend.

5. Divide half of the mixture into 12 thin, or 8-10 large, popsicle molds.

6. To release the air bubble, place the molds on the table. Fill the remaining mixture with 1/2. Then press again.

7. Push the wooden popsicle into each mold, around halfway through. Freeze for approximately three hours or until the popsicles are strong.

Set the molds in hot water for 10-20 seconds to free, and gently remove the popsicles.

Mocha Ice Cream

This milk-free ice cream reflects a delightful frozen delight. Plus, this version doesn't require an ice cream maker. Just blend and freeze is all you need to do. The xanthan gum makes the ice cream soft and rich in texture.

Serves: 6

Prep. Time: 120 minutes

Cook Time: 0 minutes Nutritional Facts Serving Size: 50 g Calories: 113

Total Fat: 11.6 g; Saturated Fat: 9.8 g; Trans Fat: 0.0 g Cholesterol: 7 mg; Sodium: 16 mg;

Potassium: 155 mg Total Carbohydrates: 4.1 g; Dietary Fiber: 1.9 g; Sugar: 1.4 g Protein: 1.4 g

Vitamin A: 1 %; Vitamin C: 2 %, Calcium: 1 %; Iron: 5 %

Ingredients:

- 1 cup of coconut lactose

- One-quarter cup heavy cream

- 2 lb Swerve/erythritol

- 15 drops of stevia-liquid

- 2 cups of cocoa powder

- 1 microwave instant coffee

- One quarter teaspoon xanthan gum

Guidelines:

1. Add all ingredients to a blender and combine until smooth and creamy.

2. Pour into an airtight box and cover with a lid.

3. 2-3 hours Freezing.

4. Serve, and have fun.

Lemon Gelato

This dairy-free treat is so delicious that you'll want to enjoy a bowlful even in the middle of winter. Also packed with vitamin C, this dessert boosts your immune system and helps keep the sniffles away.

Serves: 6

Prep. Time: 15 minutes, plus 1 hour cooling and 1 hour freezing

Cook Time: 30 minutes Nutritional

Facts Serving Size: 155 g Calories: 283

Total Fat: 28 g; Saturated Fat: 23.3 g; Trans Fat: 0.0 g Cholesterol: 140 mg; Sodium: 27 mg;

Potassium: 329 mg Total Carbohydrates: 13.2 g; Dietary Fiber: 5.5 g; Sugar: 4.3 g Protein: 4.5 g

Vitamin A: 3 %; Vitamin C: 32 %, Calcium: 3 %; Iron: 11 %

Ingredients:

- 1 Can Full-fat coconut milk
- 1 cup of milk, with no milk (almond)
- 4 Yolks of Eggs

- 1/2-3/4 cup sweetener granulated,

- 3/4 cup fresh lemon juice (2-3 lemons)

- 2 spoonfuls lemon peel, rubbed

Guidelines:

1. Whisk the yolks on the shells. Deposit back.

2. Combine the coconut milk, almond milk, and sweetener in a heavy saucepan over medium-high heat. Bring a cooler.

3. Reduce heat to small while the milk is simmering.

4. Slowly whisk the warm milk mixture into the egg yolks of the bowl, whisking the whole time.

5. Slowly pour the egg yolk mixture into the heated pan, whisking the whole time continuously.

6. Stir in the rubbed lemon peel.

7. Continue cooking the mixture on low heat, stirring until it densifies and coats the spoon back.

8. Out of heat strip. Stir in the juice of lemons.

9. Strain the mixture into a container to remove any seeds and lemon peel.

10. Put the container in the freezer or refrigerator to cool.

11. Freeze in a loaf pan or run through an ice cream maker, or use the Ziploc method, when cooled.

Ziploc method:

Pour over the mixture into a Ziploc, then freeze. Place the frozen mixture in a blender when ready to serve, and then blend until smooth.

Chocolate Chunk Avocado Ice Cream

Packed with healthy fat, avocados are easy to find and. This ice cream is sweet and rich in decadence. The chips of bitter chocolate balance out the sweetness and add a crunchy feel.

Serves: 10

Prep. Time: 240 minutes

Cook Time: 0 minutes Nutritional Facts Serving Size: 90 g Calories: 236

Total Fat: 23.3 g; Saturated Fat: 12.7 g; Trans Fat: 0.0 g Cholesterol: 8 mg; Sodium: 12 mg;

Potassium: 439 mg Total Carbohydrates: 12.8 g; Dietary Fiber: 7.6 g; Sugar: 1.3 g Protein: 4.0 g

Vitamin A: 3 %; Vitamin C: 8 %, Calcium: 3 %; Iron: 20 %

Ingredients:

- 2 Mature Avocados, Pulp

- 1 cup of coconut lactose

- One-half cup heavy cream

- 1/2 cup powdered cocoa

- 2 Vanilla Teaspoon Extract

- 1/2 cup Swerve / Powdered erythritol

- 25 drops of stevia-liquid

- 1 cup raspberry sprouts

Guidelines:

1. Mix all ingredients (except chocolate chips) in a blender, and blend until smooth.

2. Add chocolate chips now and stir well.

3. Switch to the airtight shell, cover with a lid and freeze 4-5 hours.

4. Serve, and have fun.

Avocado Chocolate Pudding Pops

These treats are a great way to get picky eaters to eat avocado as well. They're going to look like brown chocolate, so the kids don't know they have avocado and don't know they're eating well!

Serves: 10

Prep. Time: 15 minutes, plus 3 hours freezing Cook Time: 0 minutes Nutritional Facts Serving Size: 75 g Calories: 197

Total Fat: 19.8 g; Saturated Fat: 9.8 g; Trans Fat: 0.0 g Cholesterol: 0mg; Sodium: 26 mg; Potassium: 366 mg Total Carbohydrates: 9.4 g; Dietary Fiber: 6 g; Sugar: 0.7 g Protein: 2.4 g

Vitamin A: 1 %; Vitamin C: 9 %, Calcium: 2 %; Iron: 11 %

Ingredients:

- 6 spoonfuls of coconut milk, unsweetened (or almondMilk)

- 2 tablespoons coconut oil

- 2 cups of cocoa powder

- 2 Mature Avocados

- 2 ounces of unsweetened, chopped chocolate

- 1/4 Stevia extract with a teaspoon

- 1/4 cup low carbon sweetener powdered

- Vanilla extract with 1/2 teaspoon

- Season with salt

Guidelines:

1. Put the avocado into a food processor or a blender. Puree for about three to four minutes, or until smooth. When required, scrape down with a rubber spatula.

2. Add coconut milk, cocoa powder, sweetener, stevia, vanilla extract, and salt. Continue to process at low power until well blended, scraping the sides when necessary.

3. Melt the coconut oil and chocolate together in a microwaveable bowl at intervals of 30 seconds on high, stirring until it is smooth.

4. Spoon 1/2 of the mixture into Popsicle molds, press the molds to release air bubbles on a hard flat surface.

5. Spoon the remainder of the mixture into the pot. Then tap again.

6. Press wooden popsicle sticks, about 2/3 deep within the container.

7. Freeze approximately 3 hours, or until mounted.

8. Run hot water over the mold for about 30 seconds to release the popsicles. Gently twist to get released.

COOKIES

Browned Chocolate Chip Buttered Cookie

Try this delicious one-skillet recipe for a mouth-watering treat, for which your taste buds will be thankful!

Serves: 12

Prep. Time: 30 minutes Cook Time: 30 minutes Nutritional Facts Serving Size: 38 g Calories: 198

Total Fat: 16.8 g; Saturated Fat: 6.1 g; Trans Fat: 0 g Cholesterol: 36 mg; Sodium: 139 mg;

Potassium: 182 mg Total Carbohydrates: 9.5 g; Dietary Fiber: 3.2 g; Sugar: 4.8 g Protein: 4.7 g

Vitamin A: 5%; Vitamin C: 0%; Calcium:5%; Iron: 7%

Ingredients:

- 1 Grand Egg
- 1 cup of pure vanilla extract
- One and a half cup Butter
- 1/2 cup chocolate chips, free from sugar

- 1/2 tea cubit sea salt

- Splenda 1/4 cup, or natural granulated sweetener

- 2 tables of almond flour

- 2 cups of coconut sugar

Guidelines:

1. Preheat the oven to either 350F or 176C

2. Heat the butter in a 9 inch cast iron skillet until it bubbles. Reduce temperatures to low. Pan cover. Cook the butter, occasionally stirring, until browning begins. Take the skillet off heat when brown. Allow cooling for 5 minutes or so.

In the meantime, whisk together the eggs and the vanilla extract. Add the sweetener and coconut sugar. Whisk until combined. If the butter is cool, add the mixture into the egg. Combine fine.

4. Sew in the almond flour and gently press any lumps over the sieve. Add the salt and the chocolate chips in half. Mix in gently until creamy is the batter. Batter Spoon into the skillet. Top with leftover chocolate chips.

5. Heat for around 25–30 minutes or until the top is set, and when embedded into the inside, a toothpick tells the truth. Serve with frozen yogurt or ice cream with no sugar.

Chocolate Chunk Cookies

These desserts are scrumptious and will remind you of Ahoy Chips. These low-carb versions of favorite cookies from my childhood. On the outside, they're crisp, yet soft inside. Dunk as a snack, in almond or coconut milk.

Serves: 8

Prep. Time: 5 minutes Cook Time: 15 minutes Nutritional Facts Serving Size: 60 g Calories: 285

Total Fat: 27.8 g; Saturated Fat: 13.8 g; Trans Fat: 0.0g Cholesterol: 77 mg; Sodium: 107 mg;

Potassium: 282 mg Total Carbohydrates: 8.8 g; Dietary Fiber: 4.7 g; Sugar: 1.0 g Protein: 7.9 g

Vitamin A: 8 %; Vitamin C: 0 %, Calcium: 7 %; Iron: 21 %

Ingredients:

- One cup of almond flour

- 3 spoonfuls of un-aromatized whey protein

- 2 spoonfuls of coconut flour

- 8 spoonfuls of unsalted butter

- Vanilla extract with 2 teaspoons of consistency • 1/4 cup Swerve / Erythritol

- 10 drops of stevia-liquid

- Baking Powder with 1/2 teaspoon

- 2 Grand Eggs

- 1 cup slice of chocolate

Guidelines:

1. Put the eggs in a blender and blend until smooth.

2. Add butter now and stir again.

3. Add all ingredients leftover and mix well.

4. Make small, round cookies and place them in a baking platter.

5. Bake 15–20 minutes.

6. Serve, and have fun.

Chocolate Macaroon Cookies

These super easy and super yummy macaroons! Coconut and chocolate are wonderful combinations. They are delectably chewy sweet chocolate.

Serves: 10

Prep. Time: 5 minutes Cook Time: 15 minutes Nutritional Facts Serving Size: 38 g Calories: 156

Total Fat: 14.6 g; Saturated Fat: 8.4 g Trans Fat: 0.0g Cholesterol: 37 mg; Sodium: 75 mg;

Potassium: 171 mg Total Carbohydrates: 5.4 g; Dietary Fiber: 3.0 g; Sugar: 1.2 g Protein: 4.0 g

Vitamin A: 1 %; Vitamin C: 1 %, Calcium: 3 %; Iron: 12 %

Ingredients:

- One cup of almond flour

- 3 spoonfuls of coconut Flour

- 1/4 cup powdered cocoa

- 1/3 cup/erythritol

- 1 cup shredded coconut, unsweetened

- 1/4 cup of salt

- 2 Grand Eggs

- 1/4 teaspoon coconut oil

- 1 Vanilla Tablespoon Extract

Guidelines:

1. Preheat oven to 355 ° C.

2. Put all ingredients in a bowl, and thoroughly blend.

3. Make 10-12 small, round balls and transfer them to the baking platter.

4. Bake for another 15 minutes.

5. Serve, and have fun.

Turmeric Ginger Cookies

These cookies are nut-free, milk-free, flourless, and every cookie is almost sugar-free. Turmeric and ginger are powerful, widely used spices for cooking and medicinal purposes. These spices are used to treat various problems relating to digestion and the stomach. Both spices have antioxidant properties that help prevent cancerous tumors from growing

Serves: 15

Prep. Time: 15 minutes Cook Time: 10-15 minutes Nutritional Facts Serving Size: 16 g Calories: 44

Total Fat: 3.9 g; Saturated Fat: 3.2 g; Trans Fat: 0.0 g Cholesterol: 11 mg; Sodium: 60 mg;

Potassium: 50 mg Total Carbohydrates: 3.6 g; Dietary Fiber: 1.8 g; Sugar: 0.7 g Protein: 0.8 g

Vitamin A: 0 %; Vitamin C: 1 %, Calcium: 0 %; Iron: 9 %

Ingredients:

- 1 cup coconut butter, softened • 1 egg

- 1 teaspoon turmeric powder

- 1 teaspoon vanilla extract

- 1/4 cup low carb granulated sweetener

- 1/4 teaspoon baking soda

- 1/4 teaspoon sea salt

- 1/8 teaspoon black pepper, or more • 2 heaping teaspoon ginger, ground

Guidelines:

1. In a food processor, place the egg, coconut butter, and vanilla extract. Blend well when combined.

2. Stir in the baking soda, sweetener, and all the spices. Blend all over again until combined.

3. Form the mixture of cookies into 1 "balls. Place 1 "apart in a cookie sheet lined with parchment. Press to flatten each cookie into cookie forms. Do not over-spread.

4. Bake for 10-15 minutes or until slightly brown, for 350F.

5. Enable the cookies on the cookie sheet to cool down a bit. They are going to be delicate, fresh from the oven. Move on a cooling rack when slightly cool and allow to fully cool, hardening as they cool.

6. Store in an airtight container.

Remarks:

Don't completely melt the coconut butter. Just soften it. If, because the butter is too runny, the cookie dough mixture does not form into a ball, place the mixture in the refrigerator for a few minutes to make it moldable.

Wal-nutty Coconut Brownies

While milky and gluten-free, these brownies are very decadent and tasty. They are not going to taste anything like coconut. The chocolate must mask the coconut flavor. When you want lighter plates, make sure you use blanched almond flour, removing the skins. The walnuts and the shreds of coconut add a delectable flavor.

Serves: 20 minutes

Prep. Prep. Time: 15 minutes Cook Time : 30 minutes Serving Nutritional Facts Size: 49 g Calories: 234 Total Fat: 21.4 g; Saturated Fat: 12.2 g; Trans Fat: 0.0 g Cholesterol: 16 mg ; Sodium: 42 mg;

Potassium: 226 mg Total carbohydrate: 10.6 g; dietary fiber: 3.0 g ; sugar: 4.5 g

Vitamin A: 0 percent; vitamin C: 1 percent; calcium: 4 percent;

Ingredients:

- 3/4 cup powdered cocoa

- 2 teaspoons or 1/2 cup organic stevia powder extractXylitol birch (or 1/2 cup raw honey or maple syrup)

- 2 eggs

- One and a half tablespoon baking soda

- 1/2 cup, chopped walnuts

- 1/2 cup coconut shredded

- 1/2 cup coconut milk, whole, canned

- 1 Vanilla Teaspoon Extract

- 1 cup melted coconut oil

- 1 cup of almond flour, pickled

Guidelines:

1. Preheat oven 350F.

2. The eggs, chocolate, coconut milk, coconut oil, and Vanilla are mixed in a mixing pot.

3. Combine baking soda, almond flour, and shredded coconut in yet another mixing bowl.

4. Blend the two mixtures. Pour into a baking dish.

5. Bake within 30 minutes. When cooked, allow 15 minutes to cool before they serve.

CAKES

Keto Dessert with Strawberry

This baked treat is incredibly quick and straightforward to produce. All you need to do is put it all together and pop it out in the oven and 5 minutes. The delicious dessert is an excellent vitamin C source. This is also a good source of calcium, vitamin A, fiber, and protein.

Serves: 2

Prep. Time: 5 minutes Cook Time: 5 minutes Serving Size Nutritional Facts: 159 g Calories: 361

Total Fat: 33,5 g; Saturated Fat: 14,3 g; Trans Fat: 0,0 g Cholesterol: 74 mg ; Sodium: 42 mg; Potassium: 343 mg Total Carbohydrate: 12,4 g; Dietary Fiber: 4,4 g; Sugar: 4,6 g Protein: 6,8 g

Vitamin A: 14 percent; vitamin C: 71 percent; calcium: 12 percent;

Ingredients:

- 1 cup, chopped strawberries
- ½ cup almond powder
- ½ cubicle butter
- One cup of fresh whipped cream

Guidelines:

1. Preheat oven to 355 ° C.

2. Attach the strawberries, almond powder, butter, and blend in a bowl thoroughly.

3. Bake for 5 minutes and transfer to a baking dish.

4. Put on and eat whipped cream.

Mexicano Chocolate Cookies

These cookies are savory, sweet, and taste fantastic. They taste delicious that nobody would think they're dairy-free, gluten-free, and low-carb. Such snacks are very rich in chocolate and have a touch of fire.

Serves: Five

Makes: 15 Cookies. Time: 20 minutes Cook Time: 15 minutes Serving Nutritional Facts Size: 45 g Calories: 184 Total Fat: 15.1g; Saturated Fat: 11.8 g; Trans Fat: 0 g Cholesterol: 56 mg ; Sodium: 79 mg ; Potassium: 111 mg Total Carbohydrates: 10.3 g Dietary Fiber: 2.3 g ; Sugar: 7.4 g Protein: 2.7 g Vitamin A: 5%; Vitamin C: 2% Calcium: 2%; Iron: 13% Calcium: 2%

Ingredients:

• 8 teaspoons of unsweetened ground cocoa

• 4 Grand Eggs

• 3/4 cup of coconut meal

• 3 cups of salted butter

• 2 Vanilla Teaspoons

• 2 1/2 cinnamon spoons

- 1/4 cup of salt

- Cayenne pepper 1/2 teaspoons

- 1/2 tablespoon stevia oil

- One-half cup coconut oil

- 1 1/2 cups of chili powder

Guidelines:

1. Preheat to 350F on the oven.

2. Put the coconut flour in a mixing pot.

3. Add the cocoa powder, chili powder, cayenne pepper, stevia, and salt. Blend all the ingredients.

4. Put the butter and the coconut oil in a microwaveable dish.

Microwave until liquefied, for around 10-15 seconds.

5. To the butter mixture, add the eggs and Vanilla. Whisk them along.

6. For dry ingredients, add the butter mixture. Blend well with the wet ingredients, before the dry ingredients are fully soaked. Knead, if you have to, with your legs.

7. Grease a frying pan. Forme the dough into cookies with your fingertips. Do not roll, as the bits break.

8. Bake for 12-15 minutes approx. When you take them out of the oven, the cookies will be warm.

9. Let them cool down for several minutes. Treat yourself to low-carb milk

Chocolate Cupcakes

Mascarpone cheese is both textured and tastes similar to cream cheese. The cheese is also used for its faint creamy flavor in Italian desserts. Even the cheese makes those cupcakes ultra-creamy!

Serves: 12

Prep. Prep. Time: 10 minutes Cook Time: 15 minutes Serving Size Nutritional Facts: 24 g Calories: 65

Net fat: 3.8 g; 0.9 g Trans fat: 0.0 g Cholesterol: 30 mg; 24 mg sodium;

Potassium: 77 mg Total carbohydrates: 3.2 g; dietary fiber: 1.7 g;

Vitamin A: 1 percent; 0 percent vitamin C; 3 percent calcium; iron: 4 percent

Ingredients:

- 2 eggs
- Powder with ½ cup protein
- One and a half cup almond powder
- 2 ounces. Butterfly

- ¼ cup dark powdered cocoa

- 1-liter flaxseed, soil

- ¼ cup sweetening liquid

Guidelines:

1. Add eggs in a bowl, and beat until smooth.

2. For 1-2 minutes, add protein powder, almond powder, cocoa powder, liquid sweetener, mascarpone, and beat.

3. Pour this blend into molded cupcakes and bake for 15 minutes.

4. Serve, and have fun.

No-Bake Mini Lemon Tarts

These sucrose-free, egg-free, and gluten-free tarts are rare, delicious treats. These are filled with healthy fats, and they're also dairy-free if you use coconut oil. You may also opt to use a rice meal rather than a nutmeal. The nut meal gives the crust a brown color.

Serves 24 Prep. Time: 30 minutes Cook time: 0 minutes Serving Size Nutritional Facts: 30 g Calories: 128

Total fat: 12.4 g; 5.7 g Saturated fat; 0.0 g Cholesterol trans fat: 16 mg; 76 mg sodium;

Potassium: 96 mg Total carbohydrate: 3.7 g; dietary fiber: 1.9 g; protein sugar: 2.3 g

Vitamin A: 4%; Vitamin C: 4%; Calcium: 3%; Iron: 4 percent;

Ingredients:

For the crust:

- Melted 4 1/2 spoonful of butter, coconut oil or ghee

- 3/4 cup coconut, washed, rubbed finely,

- 3 cups of lemon juice

- Low carbon sweetener, equal to 2 spoonfuls of sugar

- 1 cup almond, or other cashew-like nut flour • 1 1/2 cups of vanilla extract
- Cup of salt

For the filling:

- 1 tablespoon of vanilla extract, sugar-free • 1/2 cup butter, coconut oil or ghee, softened to ambient temperature
- 1/3 cup coconut, full fat (or almond-like low-carb milk)
- 1/3 cup fresh lemon juice;
- 1/4 cup of salt
- 2 cups of lemon extract
- 2 medium lemon grated zest
- 1/4 cup low carb sweetener plus 1 tablespoon of sugar

Guidelines:

For the crust:

1. Grease 2 parts of mini-muffin pan size 12 cups.

2. Combine all the crust ingredients in a medium mixing dish until well combined.

3. Roll 2 teaspoons of the mixture of crust dough into balls then press into the prepared tart pans.

4. Chill the crusts to ready for filling.

For the filling:

1. Put the butter in a saucepan. Beat until smooth. You may also blend it in a food processor.

2. In a bowl, add the milk, sweetener, lemon juice, extracts, salt, and zest. Beat the mixture until it is solid. Then blend until smooth when using a processor.

3. Taste check. Add more lemon juice or sweetener, if needed.

Bringing the tarts together:

Spoon the filling into the crusts put together. Garnish with melon zest where needed.

2. Quiet before the filling is set.

Remarks:

If the leftover filling is available, serve it as lemon pudding is. Instead, you can place them in liners or muffin pans for the mini paper cupcake, freeze, and then serve as fat lemon bombs.

Slow Cooker Chocolate Cake

Bring this amazing dark chocolate cake in your slow cooker to use. Replace the coconut milk with full table cream for more fat.

Serves Slow Cooker 10: Prep 6-quarter. Cook Time: 20 minutes: Small 2 1/2-3 hours of Nutritional facts

Serving size: 83 g Calories: 330 Total Fat: 28.6 g; Saturated Fat: 12.9 g; Trans Fat: 0 g Cholesterol: 111 mg ; Sodium: 167 mg ; Potassium: 524 mg Total Carbohydrate: 11.6 g; Nutritional Fiber: 5.9 g ; Sugar: 2.4 g Protein: 12.8 g Vitamin A: 8%; Vitamin C: 2%; Calcium: 14%; Iron:26%

Ingredients:

• 4 Grand Eggs

• A combination of 3/4 cup sweetener • 3/4 cup almond or coconut milk, unsweetened • 2/3 cup cocoa powder

• 2 spoonfuls of baking powder

• 1/4 cup of salt

• 1/4 cup protein powder with whey, unflavored • 1/2 cup butter, melted

• 1 spoonful of vanilla extract • 1 1/2 cups of almond flour

Available as:

- 1/2 cup, sugar-free chocolate chips

Guidelines:

1. Grease the cooker until slow.

2. Whisk together the almond flour, baking powder, chocolate powder, protein powder, sweetener, and salt in a medium mixing bowl.

3. Stir in the extract of milk, eggs, butter, and Vanilla. Stir until you have combined well. If using, whisk in the chocolate chips.

4. Pour into the slow cooker, which is greased. Cook on low for 2 1/2-3 hours. Switch the slow cooker off. Let them cool down for 20-30 minutes. Cut into slices when refrigerated to a dry. Serve with whipped cream, finely topped.

Molten Lava Chocolate Cakes

This cake is fudgy with a gooey molten core. This low carb and dairy-free version also have a high iron content and a good protein source.

Serves: 2

Prep. Time: 20 minutes Cook Time: 11-12 minutes Serving Facts Size: 123 g Calories: 527 Total Fat: 54.3 g; Saturated Fat: 36.9 g; Trans Fat: 0.0 g Cholesterol: 186 mg ; Sodium: 79 mg ; Potassium: 414 mg Total Carbohydrates: 15.6 g; Dietary Fiber: 8.3 g ; Sugar: 1.1 g Protein: 12.4 g Vitamin A: 5%; Vitamin C: 0%; Calcium: 8%; Iron: 41%.

Ingredients:

• 1 cup of almond flour

• 1/4 cup coconut oil, plus ramekin grease extra)

• Vanilla extract with 1/4 teaspoon

• 2 1/5 ounces of deep, dairy-free chocolate (85%)

• 2 Grand Eggs

• 15 drops of stevia-liquid

• Powdered cocoa, to dust

Guidelines:

1. Preheat 375F for the oven.

2. Grease 2 bits of 4-ounce coconut oil ramekins and then sprinkle with cocoa powder.

3. Melt together the coconut oil and the chocolate, then apply the vanilla extract.

4. Whisk together the eggs and stevia in a big mixing cup.

5. In the egg mixture, gradually add the chocolate mixture. Beat well when combined.

6. In a bowl, add the almond flour. Mix once well installed in.

7. The batter is divided into 2 ramekins.

8. Bake for11-12 minutes. Make sure you 're not over baking.

9. Pass a knife over the ramekins' rims. Cover with a board over the ramekin. Flip the ramekin and the plate over. Lift the ramekin and dislodge the cake to the plate.

10. Let the other ramekin repeat. Serve straight away.

Smoothies

Peanut Butter Caramel Shake

This frosty coconut milkshake is flavored with peanut butter and is delightfully jazzed with salted caramel. This frozen treat represents a good source of iron and fiber.

Serves: 2

Prep. Time: 5 minutes Cook Time: 0 minutes Nutritional Facts Serving Size: 271 g Calories: 472 Total Fat: 48.2 g; Saturated Fat: 34.4 g; Trans Fat: 0.0 g Cholesterol: 31 mg; Sodium: 201 mg; Potassium: 424 mg Total Carbohydrate: 12 g; Dietary Fiber: 5.0 g; Sugar: 5.5 g Protein: 6.9 g Vitamin A: 7%; Vitamin C: 6%; Calcium: 3%; Iron: 19% Protein: 5.5 g Protein: 6.9 g Vitamin A: 7%;

Ingredients:

- 7 Cubes of ice
- 1 cup Milk coconut
- 2 cups of peanut butter
- 1 liter of maple syrup
- 2 tablespoons of salted Torani caramel

- 1/4 hp. Xanthan Chicken

Guidelines:

1. Place all ingredients in a blender and mix until smooth creamy.

Pour over in the bottle and drink.

Cocoa-Coconut- Macadamia Smoothie

This delicious smoothie is all bundled into one coffee, dessert, snack, and fat bomb. This milk-free treat is packed with good healthy fats, which will help you feel full longer.

Serves: 2

Prep. Time: 5 minutes Cook Time: 0 minutes Nutritional Information Serving size: 224 g Calories: 279 Total Fat: 28.2 g; Saturated Fat: 20.3 g; Trans Fat: 0.0 g Cholesterol: 0 mg; Sodium: 96 mg; Potassium: 313 mg Total Carbohydrate: 10.9 g; Dietary Fiber: 5.1 g; Sugar: 3.7 g Protein: 3.2 g Vitamin A: 0%; Vitamin C: 4%; Calcium: 3%; Iron: 12%.

Ingredients:

- 1 cup of ice cubes

- 1 Salt Dash

- 1 spoonful of cocoa powder, unsweetened

- Vanilla extract with 1/2 teaspoon

- 2 teaspoons of macadamia nuts, salted crushed

- 2 tablespoons Swab/erythritol or other low-carbon equivalent sugar

- 3/4 cup coconut milk, without sweetening

Guidelines:

1. Put all the ingredients into a mixer.

2. Blend until smooth and yummy.

3. Pour in 2 containers.

4. Using whipped coconut cream, macadamia nuts to top each serving, and coconut bread.

Spinach Avocado Banana Smoothie

You can enjoy this quick to make a delicious smoothie as a breakfast or as a snack drink. This smoothie is filled in nutrients that will give you the morning boost you need in only a few ingredients.

Serves: Five

Prep. Time: 3 minutes Mix Time: 2 minutes Nutritional Information Serving Size: 296 g Calories: 197 Total Fat: 8 g; Saturated Fat: 1.7 g; Trans Fat: 0 g Cholesterol: 0 mg; Sodium: 62 mg; Potassium: 367 mg; Total Carbohydrates: 13.6 g; Dietary Fiber: 3.7 g; Sugar: 7 g Protein: 20.6 g Vitamin A: 24%; Vitamin C: 16%; Calcium: 4%; Iron: 5% Protein: 20.6 g

Ingredients:

- Two cups of spinach

- 1 large, frozen banana

- Advocate 1

- 1 cup of honey

- 1 bag of gelatin or 1 scoop protein isolate

- 1 glass of Water

- Three cups of ice

Guidelines:

Put all ingredients into the mixer. Mix until smooth.

Almond Avocado Smoothie

Choosing a healthy almond butter is essential to this smoothie. By the almond butter, you choose you to get most of your flavor. Copper and calcium are present in almond butter, all of which play a crucial role in maintaining a healthy nervous system and healthy brain cells. Almond butter also contains a high proportion of vitamin E, magnesium, fiber, and balanced unsaturated fatty acids.

Serve: Plan 2. Time: 3 minutes Blend Time: 2 minutes Serving Nutritional Facts Size: 214 g Calories: 359 Total Fat: 22,2 g; Saturated Fat: 6,9 g; Trans Fat: 0 g Cholesterol: 22 mg; Sodium: 128 mg; Potassium: 437 mg Total Carbohydrates: 13,1 g; Dietary Fiber: 4 g; Sugar: 4,5 g Protein: 28,7 g Vitamin A: 6%; Vitamin C: 9%; Calcium: 18%; Iron: 6%.

Ingredients:

- 1/2 avocado, cut, washed, pitted

- Quarter and a half cup

- 1/2 cup almond unsweetened milk, coffee

- Vanilla extract with 1/2 teaspoon

- 2 scoops of Vanilla protein isolate

- 1 pound of almond butter

- Cinnamon skewer

- 1 Stevia Packet

- 2 to 4 cubes of ice

Guidelines:

1. Put everything, except the ice cubes, into a blender. Blend until it's feeling smooth.

2. Bring ice cubes in. Blend one more time.

3. Pour the bottle back. Enjoy it!

Almond Strawberry Delight

This refreshing smoothie has a creamy sweet taste and is nutty. Strawberries, besides antioxidants, also contain potassium, folate, dietary fiber, manganese. Some of the health benefits include improving the eyes and alleviating arthritis, gout, high blood pressure, and various other cardiovascular-related diseases.

Serve: Plan 2. Time: 3 minutes Blend Time: 2 minutes Nutritional Facts Serving Size: 334 g Calories: 352 Total Fat: 24.2 g Saturated Fat: 13.3 g; Trans Fat: 0 g Cholesterol: 78 mg ; Sodium: 240 mg ; Potassium: 219 mg Total Carbohydrate: 9 g; Dietary Fiber: 1.3 g ; Sugar: 5.2 g Protein: 26 g Vitamin A: 17%; Vitamin C: 12%; Calcium: 33%;

Ingredients:

- 16 ounces of unsweetened, vanilla almond milk

- 1 Stevia Packet

- Heavy cream with 4-ounces

- 2 scoops of vanilla protein isolate or 4 tablespoons of gelatin

Plus 1 Vanilla Teaspoon extract

- 1/4 cup dried, unsweetened strawberries

Guidelines:

1. Throw it all into a blender. Mix in until smooth. Pour in a glass. Enjoy it!

Creamy Blackberry

This delicious smoothie drink is packed with anthocyanins, compounds that help keep the heart safe. Blackberry fiber and magnesium also promote strong blood flow and avoid blockage of the arteries, reducing the risk of strokes and heart attacks.

Serve: 2 Prep. Time: 3 minutes Mix Time: 2 minutes Serving Nutritional Facts Size: 268 g Calories: 300 Total Fat: 17 g; Saturated Fat: 10,4 g; Trans Fat: 0 g Cholesterol: 62 mg; Sodium: 76 mg ; Potassium: 156 mg Total Carbohydrate: 12,2 g; Dietary Fiber: 3,8 g; Sugar: 7,6 g Protein: 25,9 g Vitamin A: 16%; Vitamin C: 26%; Calcium: 7%; Iron: 4%.

Ingredients:

• Fresh, 1 cup blackberries

• 1 Stevia Packet

• 3/4 cup heavy cream with whipping

• 2 scoops of vanilla protein isolate or 4 tablespoons of gelatin plus 2 Vanilla Teaspoon Extract

• 1 cup of ice cube

Guidelines:

1. Put everything, except the ice cubes, into a blender. Mix in until smooth.

2. Bring ice cubes in. Blend one more time.

3. Pour the bottle back. Enjoy it!

Cream Chocolate Milkshake

This is a quick and easy way to make your keto-friendly milkshake in chocolate. This low carb version is delicious, but you can enjoy it guilt-free because you can eat a lot of fat!

Serves: 2

Prep. Time: 3 minutes Blend Time: 2 minutes Nutritional Facts Serving Size: 361 g Calories: 120 Total Fat: 24.2 g; Saturated Fat: 13.3 g; Trans Fat: 0 g Cholesterol: 78 mg ; Sodium: 214 mg ; Potassium: 218 mg Total Carbohydrate: 7.4 g; Nutritional Fiber: 0.9 g ; Sugar: 4.1 g Protein: 14.1 g Vitamin A: 17%; Vitamin C: 1% Calcium: 32%; Iron: 5% Calcium: 32%;

Ingredients:

- 16 ounces of unsweetened, vanilla almond milk
- Heavy cream, 4 ounces
- 1 scoop of protein insulating chocolate
- 1 Stevia Packet
- One and a half cup broken ice

Guidelines:

1. Put everything, except the ice cubes, into a blender. Blend until it was feeling smooth.

2. Add in the cubes of ice. Blend one more time.

3. Pour the bottle back. Enjoy it!

Hazelnut Coffee Smoothie

This smoothie blends hazelnut taste and coffee into a delicious dessert, starting the day off with a good bang!

Serves: 1 File. Time: 3 minutes Blend Time: 2 minutes Nutritional Facts Serving size: 286 g Calories: 19 Total Fat: 20.6 g; Saturated Fat: 9.6 g; Trans Fat: 0 g Cholesterol: 55 mg ; Sodium: 20 mg ; Potassium: 210 mg Total Carbohydrates: 2.7 g; Dietary Fiber: 0.9 g ; Sugar: 0 g Protein: 2.5 g Vitamin A: 12%; Vitamin C: 1% Calcium: 4%; Iron: 3% Calcium: 4%;

Ingredients:

- One-third cup heavy cream
- 1 cup coffee, cold
- 1-2 lb hazelnut syrup, sugar-free
- A cube of ice

Guidelines:

1. Put everything, except the ice cubes, into a blender—blend until smooth.

2. Bring ice cubes in. Blend one more time.

3. Pour the bottle back. Enjoy it!

The Peanut Milkshake

Peanut butter is something other than lunch for your kid! High in healthy oils and protein, this adaptable spread guides weight reduction, diabetes, and Alzheimer's sickness. Peanuts additionally contain fiber for a protected solid discharge, muscle, and bone wellbeing magnesium.

Serves: 2

Prep, Time: 3 minutes Blend Time: 2 minutes Nutritional Facts Serving Size: 326 g Calories: 278 Total Fat: 24.1 g; Saturated Fat: 14.5 g; Trans Fat: 0 g Cholesterol: 0 mg ; Sodium: 176 mg ; Potassium: 361 mg Total Carbohydrate: 11.7 g; Dietary Fiber: 2.8 g ; Sugar: 7.8 g Protein: 5.9 g Vitamin A: 0 percent; Vitamin C: 3 percent Calcium: 16 percent; Iron: 16 percent

Ingredients:

• 2 cups of peanut butter, all-natural

• Extract 1 tsp Vanilla

• 1 Stevia Packet

• 1 cup almond milk, coffee

• 1/2 tablespoon coconut milk, standard

• 1 cup of ice cubes

Guidelines:

1. Put everything, except the ice cubes, into a blender—blend until smooth.

2. Bring ice cubes in. Blend one more time. Pour the bottle back. Enjoy it!

Vanilla Chocolate Spice Shake

This smoothie is a delicious gourmet treat. With the unexpected touch of cayenne fire, this cool blend is spiced up. Cayenne is a spice notorious for neutralizing acidity and stimulating circulation. This makes it a well-known ingredient in purifying and detoxifying regimes.

Serves: 2

Prep. Time: 3 minutes Blend Time: 2 minutes Nutritional Facts Serving Size: 171 g Calories: 218 Total Fat: 22.6 g; Saturated Fat: 18.7 g; Trans Fat: 0 g Cholesterol: 0 mg ; Sodium: 10 mg ; Potassium: 246 mg Total Carbohydrate: 5.8 g; Dietary Fiber: 3.3 g ; Sugar: 1.2 g Protein: 2.3 g Vitamin A: 1%; Vitamin C: 2%; Calcium: 2%.

Ingredients:

• One-quarter cup coconut cream

• 1/2 to 1 cup of Water

• Pinch 1/2 cayenne powder

• Chia seeds or 1 tbsp flax seeds

• 2 tbsp of unsweetened powdered cocoa

• 2 tbsp of unwashed coconut oil

- Vanilla splash extract

- Ground pick cinnamon

- Ice cubes, if you wish

Guidelines:

1. Bring all, except the ice cubes, into a blender. Mix in until smooth.

2. Put in the cubes of ice. Blend one more time.

3. Pour the bottle back. Love it!

Heavenly Creamy Chocolate Shake

Whipping cream makes the shake light as creamy and airy. This exciting beverage is also high out of this planet, is calcium.

Serves: 1

Prep. Time: 3 minutes Blend Time: 2 minutes Serving Nutritional Facts Size: 306 g Calories: 236 Total Fat: 19 g; Saturated Fat: 10 g; Trans Fat: 0 g Cholesterol: 55 mg ; Sodium: 197 mg ; Potassium: 305 mg Total Carbohydrate: 14.3 g; Dietary Fiber: 2.8 g ; Sugar: 8.4 g Protein: 2.9 g Vitamin A: 12%; Vitamin C: 0%; Calcium: 33%; Iron: 8%.

Ingredients:

• 1 cup of almond milk, unsweetened

• 1/3 cup heavy cream with whipping

• 1 Stevia Packet

• Vanilla extract with 1/2 teaspoon

• 1 tablespoon of unsweetened ground cocoa

• Trois cubes of ice

Guidelines:

1. Bring all, except the ice cubes, into a blender. Blend until feeling smooth.

2. Put ice cubes in. Blend one more time.

3. Pour the bottle back. Love it!

Creamy Avocado Chocolate Smoothie

The avocado makes for a sinfully delicious drink in this smoothie. Rich, smooth and creamy, and velvety. The avocado also packs a healthy amount of good fats into this drink.

Serves: 2

Prep. Time: 3 minutes Blend Time: 2 minutes Serving Nutritional Facts Size: 286 g Calories: 450 Total Fat: 32,3 g; Saturated Fat: 12,1 g; Trans Fat: 0 g Cholesterol: 42 mg ; Sodium: 53 mg ; Potassium: 535 mg; Total Carbohydrate: 16,6 g; Dietary Fiber: 6,9 g; Sugar: 7,2 g Protein: 26,9 g Vitamin A: 12%; Vitamin C: 17%; Calcium: 6%; Iron: 6%

Ingredients:

- 1 Frozen Avocado
- One-half cup heavy cream
- 1 pound of dark chocolate
- 1 Splenda Teaspoon
- 1 bag of gelatin or 1 scoop of protein-coated with chocolate
- 1 glass of Water

Guidelines:

Place all ingredients into the mixer. Mix in until smooth

Peach Coconut Smoothie

Fresh peaches in the summer and coconut milk make this a sweet, creamy, dairy-free combination. Using chilled coconut milk gives it a consistency which is like a milkshake. With the high amount of good fats, coconut milk also makes it extra rich and creamy.

Serves: 2

Prep. Time: 3 minutes Mix Time: 2 minutes Serving Nutritional Facts Size: 342 g Calories: 399 Total Fat: 28.8 g; Saturated Fat: 25.4 g; Trans Fat: 0 g Cholesterol: 0 mg ; Sodium: 76 mg ; Potassium: 464 mg; Total Carbohydrate: 13.9 g; Dietary Fiber: 3.8 g ; Sugar: 10.2 g Protein: 27.4 g Vitamin A: 5%; Vitamin C: 16%; Calcium: 4%; Iron: 14%;

Ingredients:

- 1 1/2 frozen peaches,
- 1 cup of coconut lactose
- 1 mp. Zest Lemon
- 2 Gelatin packs
- 1 Top Ice

Guidelines:

Place all ingredients into the mixer. Mix until smooth.

Strawberry Coconut-Smoothie

This dairy-free smoothie has only 5 ingredients and is creamy and sweet. The Vanilla makes a taste like ice cream to this blend. After blending for added flavor, I love to add a little unsweetened shredded coconut.

Serves: 1

Prep. Time: 3 minutes Blend Time: 2 minutes Serving Size Nutritional facts: 219 g Calories: 438

Total Fat: 31 g; Saturated Fat: 25,7 g; Trans Fat: 0 g Cholesterol: 0 mg ; Sodium: 76 mg ; Potassium: 475 mg; Total Carbohydrate: 13,8 g Dietary Fiber: 5,7 g; Sugar: 7,6 g Protein: 28,4 g Vitamin A: 0%; Vitamin C: 64% Calcium: 5%; Iron: 25% Vitamin A: 0%

Ingredients:

- 5 Frozen Strawberries

- 1 cup of uncooked coconut milk

- 1 pound of ground flax seed

- 1 bag of gelatin or 1 scoop protein isolate

- 1 Vanilla Tablespoon Extract

Guidelines:

Place all ingredients into the mixer. Mix until smooth.

Coconut Chocolate Tofu Power Smoothie

This high fat, high protein smoothie tastes like a milkshake made from chocolate. The tofu makes the silky smoothie smooth, almost like pudding. This beverage is a delicious way to start the day!

Serves: 1

Prep. Time: 3 minutes Mix Time: 2 minutes Serving Size Nutritional facts: 395 g Calories: 401

Total Fat: 25.4 g; Saturated Fat: 18.7 g; Trans Fat: 0 g Cholesterol: 0 mg ; Sodium: 88 mg ; Potassium: 488 mg; Total Carbohydrate: 13.6 g Dietary Fiber: 4.7 g ; Sugar: 7.6 g Vitamin A: 0%; Vitamin C: 4%; Calcium: 29%; Iron: 25%

Ingredients:

• 80 ml of unbeatable coconut milk

• Tofu 1/2 cup, silken

• 1 tablespoon of unsweetened ground cocoa

• Water: 150 ml

• 1 Stevia Packet

• 1 bag of gelatin or 1 scoop protein isolate

Guidelines:

1. Place all ingredients into the mixer. Mix until smooth.

28 DAYS PLAN

Week 1

Our main objective here, at first, is to remain very plain. Simplicity is important in my mind for someone who is just starting a low carb diet. You don't want this to be a tough change (kitchen-wise), because even getting rid of your cravings would be hard. Leftovers will be another matter that we will take into account.

It is easier for you, but why put yourself through the hassle of more than once cooking the same food? Breakfast is something that I usually do in the leftover form, so I don't have to think about it in the morning, and I don't have to sweat it.

Take some food out of the refrigerator, packed for me, and where headaches, fogginess of the brain, exhaustion, and the like will make the body rile. Are you sure it's you? The first ketosis symptoms are known as the "keto flu" that drinks a ton of ad out of the door. Dowaterand eating plenty of salt, it doesn't get any easier than that. The ketogenic diet is a natural diuretic, and you're going to pee beyond normal.

Considering that you're peeing out electrolytes and you can say you're going to get a thumping headache in no time. It is really necessary to keep your salt intake and water intake high enough to re-hydrate and re-supply your electrolytes. Doing that will relieve the headaches if not absolutely, get rid of them. Drink Water with a salt sprinkling in it, if you need to. Only keep drinking water (I recommend 4 liters a day), and continue to consume salt. Trust me. It will help. If you are concerned about the salt and high blood pressure, don't be! The latest findings suggest that sodium consumption and blood pressure aren't as associated as we once thought.

Breakfast.

You want to do something simple, convenient, tasty for breakfast, and of course, it gives you leftovers. I suggest you start your weekend on day one. That way, you can make something that will last you all week long. The first week applies to convenience. Nobody wants to have breakfast before work, and we will not do that either!

Lunch.

Here too, we'll keep it easy. Most of the time, it'll be salad and meat, slathered in high-fat dressings, and calling it a day. Here we don't wish to get too rowdy. You can use the leftover meat from previous nights or conveniently accessible chicken/fish canned. Try reading the labels if you are using processed meats to find the one that contains the least (or no) additives!

Dinner.

Dinner will be a combination of leafy greens with some meat (normally broccoli and spinach). We're going to go up on the fat again and moderate on the protein. The first 2 weeks have been no dessert.

Shopping List for Week 1

Meat

Bacon

Canned Chicken

Chicken Sausage

Chicken Thighs

Eggs

Ground Beef

Shrimp

Stew Meat

Fats

Bottle Olive Oil

Unsalted Butter (Grass-fed)

Coconut Oil

Half n' Half

Heavy Cream

Pecans

Sauces

Beef Broth

Chicken Stock

Coconut Milk

Dijon Mustard

Ranch Dressing (Full Fat)

Red Wine

Soy SauceTomato Paste

Tomato Sauce

Worcestershire

Cheese

Cheddar Cheese (Full Fat)

Parmesan Cheese

Queso Fresco Cheese

Vegetables

1 Green Pepper,

3 Onions

6 Lemons

Broccoli

Cauliflower

Green Beans

Orange

Parsley

Spinach (lots of this)

Spices

Allspice

Bay Leaf

Black Pepper

Cardamom

Cayenne Pepper

Chili Powder

ChivesCoconut Flour

Coriander

Cumin

Ginger

Minced Garlic

Onion Powder

Oregano

Paprika

Red Pepper Flakes

Salt

Xanthan Gum

Yellow Curry Powder

Day 1

Breakfast

Frittata Muffins [2 Muffins]

410 Calories, 32.3 g Fats, 2.5 g Net Carbs, and 27.3 g Protein per serving.

Lunch

Chicken Canned & Spinach Salad [2 Spinach Cups, 3 Tbsp. Olive Oil & Cup 1/3 Canned Chicken]

450 Calories, 44 g Fats, 0.5 g Net Carbs, and 13.5 g Protein per serving

Dinner

Inside out Bacon Burger [1 1/2 Patties] [Leftovers Refrigerate]

Red Pepper [Add 1 Tbsp. Butter [butter]

641 Calories, 52.5 g Fats, 4.7 g Net Carbs, and 37 g Protein per serving.

Totals for the day

1601 Calories, Fats 139.8 g, Net Carbs 7.7 g, and Protein 77.8 g

Day 2

Breakfast

Cheesy Scrambled Eggs

453 Calories, 43 g Fats, 1.2 g Net Carbs, and 19 g Protein per serving.

Lunch

Bacon Burger & Spinach Salad Leftover Inside

[4 Spinach tassels, 4 Tbsp. Olive & 3 Tbsp. Residual Meat]

624 Calories, 63.9 g Fats, 1.2 g Net Carbs, and 10.8 g Protein per serving.

Dinner

Cinnamon & Orange Beef Stew [Eat Whole Stew 80 percent]

519 Calories, 35.6 g Fats, 4.1 g Net Carbs, and 42.8 g Protein per serving.

Totals for the day

1596 Calories, 142.5 g of fats, 6.5 g of Net Carbs and 72.6 g of protein

Day 3

Breakfast

Frittata Muffins [2 Muffins]

410 Calories, 32.3 g Fats, 2.5 g Net Carbs, and 27.3 g Protein per serving.

Lunch

Quick Spinach (No Meat) Salad

[4 Spinach's Cups & 4 Tbsp. Olive oil: Olive oil]

537 Calories, 57 g Fats, 1 g Net Carbs, and

Dinner

Curry Rubbed Thigh Chicken [1 Thigh Chicken]

Fresco Fried Queso [1/4 Lb Fried Queso]

657 Calories, 44.7 g Fats, 0.6 g Net Carbs, and 40.3 g Protein per serving.

Totals for the day

1604 Calories, 134 g of fats, 4.1 g of Net Carbs and 72.6 g of protein

Day 4

Breakfast

Scrambled Fried Eggs

453 Calories, 43 g Fats, 1.2 g Net Carbs, and 19 g Protein per serving.

Lunch

Residual Rub Chicken & Spinach Salad

[4 Spinach tassels, 4 Tbsp. Olive oil & 1/3 cup chicken leftovers]

586 Calories, 58 g Fats, 1 g Net Carbs, and 15 g Protein per serving

Dinner

Chicken & Bacon Sausage Stir Fry [Freeze] [Eat 1/3 of the Full Recipe]

Residues as 2 servings] [Add 1/4 cup shredded Cheddar cheese]

541 Calories, 38.3 g Fats, 8.3 g Net Carbs, and 42.7 g Protein per serving.

Totals for the day

1580 Calories, 140 g of fats, 10.5 g of Net Carbs and 76.7 g of protein

Day 5

Breakfast

Frittata Muffins [2]

410 Calories, 32.3 g Fats, 2.5 g Net Carbs, and 27.3 g Protein per serving.

Lunch

Leftover Sausage Chicken & Spinach Salad

[4 Spinach tassels, 2 Tbsp. Stir Fry Olive Oil & Leftover Sausage (1/2 portion)

742 Calories, 70.2 g Fats, 4.7 g Net Carbs, and 20.8 g Protein per serving.

Dinner

Curry [Eat 1/6 of Total Recipe] [Freeze Leftovers as

5 Portions: 5 Portions]

[Write 1 Tbsp. Cottage oil]

451 Calories, 33.5 g Fats, 5.6 g Net Carbs, and 27.4 g Protein per serving.

Totals for the day

1602 Calories, 136 g of fats, 12.8 g of net carbs, 75.5 g of protein

Day 6

Breakfast

Scrambled Fried Eggs

453 Calories, 43 g Fats, 1.2 g Net Carbs, and 19 g Protein per serving.

Lunch

Canned Spinach & Chicken Salad

[2 Spinach tassels, 2 Tbsp. Olive oil & 1/3 cup chicken leftovers]

351 Calories, 31 g Fats, 0.5 g Net Carbs, and 15.5 g Protein per serving.

Dinner

Chorizo & Cheddar Meatballs [Freeze Leftovers] [Eat 5 Meatballs]

Pecan Roasted Green Beans [Eat 1/6 Total Recipe] [SaveResidues as 5 Portions]

798 Calories, 63 g Fats, 7.1 g Net Carbs, and 40.2 g Protein per serving.

Totals for the day

1602 Calories, 137 g of fats, 8.8 g of Net Carbs and 74.7 g of protein

Day 7

Breakfast

Scrambled Fried Eggs

[Write 1 Tbsp. Butter-extra]

553 Calories, 54 g Fats, 1.2 g Net Carbs, and 19 g Protein per serving.

Lunch

Cheese Cream & Spinach Salad

[4 Spinach tassels, 3 Tbsp. Olive oil, and 1 oz. Cheese sauce]

496 Calories, 51 g Fats, 2 g Net Carbs, and 5 g Protein per serving

Dinner

Not Chili [Eat 1/4 of Total Recipe] by Your Caveman [Freeze Leftovers as 3 Portions]

Bacon Infused Sugar Snap Peas [Save Leftovers as 2 Portions] [Eat 1/3 of the Total Recipe]

545 Calories, 31.1 g Fats, 9.6 g Net Carbs, and 53.1 g Protein per serving.

Totals for the day

1594 Calories, Fats 136.1 g, Net Carbs 12.8 g, and Protein 77.1g

Week 2

Wow, you are finishing week one. I hope you 're still having a proper diet, and finding it pretty easy to keep track of everything!

We'll be keeping it easy for breakfast again this week. We must launch a bulletproof coffee. In your coffee, it's a combination of coconut oil, butter, and heavy cream. If that repels you-and I know some of you will say "WHAT? " - Just put some faith in me! The concoction isn't as gross as it sounds. Butter is made from milk, after all. And when you put the sugar, butter, and cream together, it just adds to your coffee a decadent luxury that I'm sure you're going to like!

Breakfast.

We are going to mix things up a little for breakfast. Here's where we get bulletproof coffee added. Okay, don't misunderstand me-I know some of you won't like it. If you aren't a coffee addict, then try tea. If you're not a taste fan (which is very rare), try to make a mixture of the ingredients by yourself and eat it this way.

But why, bulletproof coffee?

The Lack of Fat. Plain and basic, the intake of medium-chain triglycerides (MCT) has been shown to result in greater losses in both animal and human adipose tissue (fat tissue). Fats!- Fats! Need I even describe this one? It has been shown that consuming fat results in greater quantities of energy, more efficient use of resources, and more significant weight loss. It's the key component of the diet, not to mention.

More Energy. Studies have shown that the rapid oxidation rate of medium-chain fatty acids (MCFAs) contributes to an increase in energy outlay. MCFAs are mainly transformed into ketones (our best friends), processed differently in the body instead of standard oils, and give us more energy overall. If you're not the biggest fan of the flavor, feel free to add sweetener and spices to this. Cinnamon, stevia, extract Vanilla. Everything you like is a nice tasting. Every day you can even turn the taste so you won't get bored! If this is your first time drinking bulletproof coffee, I suggest that you take 1-2 hours to drink it. Normally when people have a large exposure to coconut oil and are not used to it, it can often cause them to go to the bathroom. Make sure you develop coconut oil tolerance before you drink it within a 20-minute time frame.

Lunch.

We're still here to keep simple. We can incorporate more meat from the previous cooking night into every lunch that we do. Green vegetables and dressings high in fat (or vinaigrettes) are essential. Ensuring that the fats are matched with the protein quantities is very critical.

Dinner.

Dinner, again, is going to be rather simplistic. Flesh, vegetables, high-fat dressings are the foundation of our lives. Perhaps even a slathering of butter on our fruits, as we get more frisky. Don't think things over in the first 2 weeks; success is easy.

S. No dessert for this week either, but next week we're going to be delving into that!

Shopping List for Week 2

Meat

Chicken Breast

Chorizo Sausage

Sauces/Liquids

Apple Cider Vinegar

Coffee

Hot Sauce

Yellow Mustard

Crunch

Almonds

Pecans

Pork Rinds

Cheese

Blue Cheese Crumbles

Cream Cheese

Mozzarella Cheese

Vegetables

Green Beans

LemonsMushrooms

Spring Onion

Sugar Snap Peas

Spices

Baking Powder

Baking Soda

Mrs. Dash Table Blend

Tone's Southwest Chipotle Seasoning

Specialty Items

Almond Flour

Milled Flax Seed

Day 8

Breakfast

Bulletproof Coffee

273 Calories, 30 g Fats, 1 g Net Carbohydrates, and 0 g Protein per serving

Lunch

Canned Spinach & Chicken Salad

[4 Spinach tassels, 2 Tbsp. Olive oil & Surplus 2/3 Cup or Canned Chicken]

416 Calories, 32 g Fats, 1 g Net Carbs, and 27 g Protein per serving

Dinner

Chorizo Leftover Meatballs [Eat 6 Meatballs]

Pecan Roasted Green Beans [One Portion] [Use Leftovers]

921 Calories, 72.2 g Fats, 7.9 g Net Carbs, and 47.5 g Protein per serving.

Totals for the day

1610 Calories, 134.2 g of fats, 9.9 g of Net Carbs and 74.5 g of protein

Day 9

Breakfast

Bulletproof Coffee

273 Calories, 30 g Fats, 1 g Net Carbohydrates, and 0 g Protein per serving

Lunch

Cheddar Mug Cake, Chive & Bacon

573 Calories, 55 g Fats, 5 g Net Carbs and 24 g Protein per serving

Dinner

Leftover Shrimp & Cauliflower Curry [Double Serving] [Use Residues] [Add Residues]

1 TB. Butter-extra]

661 Calories, 39 g Fats, 11.2 g Net Carbs, and 54.8 g Protein per serving.

Totals for the day

1607 Calories, 135 g of fats, 17.2 g of net carbon and 78.8 g of protein

Day 10

Breakfast

Bulletproof Coffee

273 Calories, 30 g Fats, 1 g Net Carbohydrates, and 0 g Protein per serving

Lunch

Keto-Friendly Taco Tartlets [Freeze / Store Leftovers] [Eat 2 Tartlets]

481 Calories, 38.8 g Fats, 5.47 g Net Carbs, and 26.2 g Protein per serving.

Dinner

Curry Rub Chicken Thighs [Eat 2 Total Chicken Thighs] [You need to make 1 Lunch Tomorrow Extra Chicken Thigh]

Green Spinach Salad with Pepper

763 Calories, 57.8 g Fats, 4.8 g Net Carbs, and 50.3 g Protein per serving.

Totals for the day

1577 Calories, Fats 133.5 g, Net Carbs 11.2 g, and Protein 76.4g

Day 11

Breakfast

Bulletproof Coffee

273 Calories, 30 g Fats, 1 g Net Carbohydrates, and 0 g Protein per serving

Lunch

Leftover Thigh Chicken & Spinach Salad

[4 Spinach tassels, 2 Tbsp. Olive Oil & 1 Thigh Leftover Chicken]

553 Calories, 47.9 g Fats, 1.6 g Net Carbs, and 24.1 g Protein per serving.

Dinner

Strips of Buffalo Chicken [Eat 1/3 of Full Recipe] [Refigerate 2 Strips, Leftovers to Freeze]

Snap peas Bacon Infused Sugar [Eat 1 serving]

750 Calories, 58.7 g Fats, 9.1 g Net Carbs, and 42.3 g Protein per serving.

Totals for the day

1577 Calories, Fats 136.5 g, Net Carbs 11.8 g, and Protein 66.5g

Day 12

Breakfast

Bulletproof Coffee

273 Calories, 30 g Fats, 1 g Net Carbohydrates, and 0 g Protein per serving

Lunch

Sliders on Chicken Strip [Save Almond Buns]

625 Calories, 51 g Fats, 4.3 g Net Carbs, and 34.8 g Protein per serving.

Dinner

[Eat 1/2 Full Recipe] [Refrigerate Leftovers] Omnivore Burger with Creamed Spinach and Almonds

Add 1 Tbsp of Almond Flax Slider Bun [Use Leftovers]. Butter to Almond Flax Slider Bun] 773 Calories, 59.9 g Fat, 5.3 g Net Carbs, and 49.1 g Protein

Totals for the day

1671 Calories, 140.8 g Fat, 10.6 g Net Carb, and 83.9 g Protein

Day 13

Breakfast

Bulletproof Coffee

273 Calories, 30 g Fats, 1 g Net Carbohydrates, and 0 g Protein per serving

Lunch

Omnivore Burger & Salad with Spinach

[4 Spinach tassels, 2 Tbsp. Olive oil & 1/2 Omnivore Burger leftovers]

510 Calories, 42 g Fats, 2.4 g Net Carbs, and 25.9 g Protein per serving.

Dinner

Bacon Mozzarella Meatballs [5 Freeze Leftovers]

Pecan Roasted Green Beans [Eat 1 serving] [Use Leftovers]

821 Calories, 63.8 g Fats, 6.7 g Net Carbs, and 54 g Protein per serving.

Totals for the day

1605 Calories, Fats 135.8 g, Net Carbs 10.2 g, and Protein 79.9g

Day 14

Breakfast

Bulletproof Coffee

273 Calories, 30 g Fats, 1 g Net Carbohydrates, and 0 g Protein per serving

Lunch

Mozzarella Leftover Meatballs & Spinach Salad

[4 Spinach tassels, 2 Tbsp. Butter (No Olive Oil) & 4 Meatballs Leftover]

641 Calories, 51.2 g Fats, 3 g Net Carbs, and 35.2 g Protein per serving

Dinner

Stir Fry Chicken & Bacon Sausage [Eat 1 serving] [Use Leftovers]

[Add 1/4 Cup Cheddar Shredded Cheese & 1 Tbsp. Butter [butter]

641 Calories, 49.3 g Fats, 8.3 g Net Carbs, and 42.7 g Protein per serving.

Totals for the day

1555 Calories, Fats 130.5 g, Net Carbs 12.4 g, and Protein 77.9g

Week 3

We're adding a slightly fast approach this week. In the morning, we will get full of fats and fast until dinner time. There are not only a few health advantages of this, but our eating routine (and the cooking routine) is also smoother. I recommend you eat your breakfast (rather, drink) at 7 am and then eat dinner at 7 pm. Holding in between your 2 meals for 12 hours.

This will help to put your body in a state of affliction. In a fasting state, our bodies can break down extra fat stored for the energy they need. Our body is already imitating a fasting state while we are in ketosis, being that we have little or no glucose in our bloodstream, so we use the fats in our body as energy. Intermittent fasting follows the same logic-we use our stored fat instead of using the fats we consume to obtain energy.

You might think it's fantastic-you might just be able to fast and lose weight. You have to bear in mind that later you will need to eat extra fat to keep you out of a state of starvation mode. There are a variety of demonstrated benefits that come from intermittent fasting. These include blood lipid rates, durability, and the much-needed mental level clearness. If you find you can't make a quick move, then no big deal. Go back to week 1, and try as you see fit. As long as it fits into your macros, you can eat what you want. This is where things get more fun-less to think about, more cooking delight!

Breakfast.

With breakfast, we are going full-on fats just as we did last week. Every time we 're going to double the amount of bulletproof coffee (or tea), we 're drinking, which means we are doubling the amount of coconut oil, butter, and heavy cream. It is expected to come up with quite many calories, which will probably keep us full for dinner. Remember to keep on drinking water like a fiend to make sure that you stay hydrated.

Lunch.

Oh no, no lunch! Don't worry-the morning fats should keep you feeling full and energized throughout the lunch. Normally people start to hit a wall around 2 pm at first, so make sure you have plenty of water to drink, drink and drink.

Dinner.

Okay, dinner remains the same. Meats, vegetables, and fats will almost always be the standard for dinnertime. But don't worry-we're going to mix things in some bready stuff! Because guess what, this week we get to enjoy the cake! Yeah, yeah! We're going to make some low carb and fantastic degustations that will always reward you so much.

Fasts. Sweets, gourmet treatments, and weight loss – lucky us, right?

Shopping List for Week 3

Meat

Boneless, Skinless Chicken Thigh

Pork Tenderloin

Sauces

Liquid Smoke

Pesto Sauce

Red Wine Vinegar

Red Boat Fish Sauce (or Gluten-Free Fish Sauce)

Spicy Brown Mustard

Cheese

Halloumi Cheese (Mozzarella can be substituted)

Vegetables

Lemons

Spices

Dried Rosemary

Dried Sage

Ground Clove

Nutmeg

Vanilla ExtractSpeciality Items

Erythritol

Liquid Stevia

Day 15

Breakfast

Bulletproof Coffee [Double Serving]

546 Calories, 60 g Fats, 1.5 g Net Carbs, and 0 g Protein per serving.

Lunch

Fast through lunch, make sure you have plenty of water to drink!

Dinner

Pesto Chicken Roulade [Eat Whole Recipe]

[1/4 Pound Queso] Fried Queso

[Add a Spinach 4 Cups]

886 Calories, 55.8 g Fats, 3.5 g Net Carbs, and 75.5 g Protein per serving.

Dessert

Vanilla Latte Cookie [Eat 1 Cookie]

167 Calories, 17.1 g Fats, 1.4 g Net Carbs and 3.9 g Protein per Serving

Totals for the day

1599 Calories, Fats 132.9 g, Net Carbs 6.4 g, and Protein 79.4 g

Day 16

Breakfast

Bulletproof [Double serving] Coffee

546 Calories, 60 g Fats, 1.5 g Net Carbs, and 0 g Protein per serving.

Lunch

Fast through lunch, make sure you have plenty of water to drink!

Dinner

Not Chili [Eat 1 1/3 portion] of Your Caveman [Use Leftovers]

531 Calories, 23.7 g Fats, 7 g Net Carbs, and 69 g Protein.

Dessert

Cookies on Vanilla Latte [Eat 3 Cookies]

501 Calories, 51.3 g Fats, 4.3 g Net Carbs, and 11.7 g Protein per serving.

Totals for the day

1578 Calories, 135 g of fats, 12.8 g of net carbon and 80.7 g of protein

Day 17

Breakfast

Bulletproof [Double serving] Coffee

546 Calories, 60 g Fats, 1.5 g Net Carbs, and 0 g Protein per serving.

Lunch

Fast through lunch, make sure you have plenty of water to drink!

Dinner

Quick Keto BBQ Pulled Chicken [Freeze Leftovers] [Eat 1/4 Recipe]

Green Spinach Salad with Pepper

756 Calories, 50 g Fats, 6.3 g Net Carbs, and 62.5 g Protein per serving

Dessert

Cookies on Vanilla Latte [Eat 2 Cookies]

334 Calories, 34.2 g Fats, 2.8 g Net Carbs, and 7.8 g Protein per serving.

Totals for the day

1636 Calories, Fats 144.2 g, Net Carbs 10.6 g, and Protein 70.3g

Day 18

Breakfast

Bulletproof [Double serving] Coffee

546 Calories, 60 g Fats, 1.5 g Net Carbs, and 0 g Protein per serving.

Lunch

Fast through lunch, make sure you have plenty of water to drink!

Dinner

Within Bacon Burger [3 Complete Patties] [290 g of beef used]

866 Calories, 69 g Fats, 2.3 g Net Carbs, and 58 g Protein per serving.

Dessert

[Eat 1 Spice Cake] Low Carb Spice Cake

283 Calories, 27 g Fats, 3.3 g Net Carbs, and 7.3 g Protein per serving.

Totals for the day

1694 Calories, 156 g of fats, 7.1 g of net Carbs, 65.3 g of protein

Day 19

Breakfast

Bulletproof [Double serving] Coffee

546 Calories, 60 g Fats, 1.5 g Net Carbs, and 0 g Protein per serving.

Lunch

Fast through lunch, make sure you have plenty of water to drink!

Dinner

The explosion of Cheddar Bacon [Eat 1/3 of Recipe] [Refrigerate Leftovers as 2

Portions] Portions: Portions

720 Calories, 63.7 g Fats, 4.9 g Net Carbs, and 54.7 g Protein per serving.

Dessert

[Eat 1 Spice Cake] Low Carb Spice Cake

283 Calories, 27 g Fats, 3.3 g Net Carbs, and 7.3 g Protein per serving.

Totals for the day

1549 Calories, 150.7 g of fats, 9.7 g of net Carbs and 62 g of protein

Day 20

Breakfast

Bulletproof [Double serving] Coffee

546 Calories, 60 g Fats, 1.5 g Net Carbs, and 0 g Protein per serving.

Lunch

Fast through lunch, make sure you have plenty of water to drink!

Dinner

Bacon-Wrapped Pork Tenderloin [Eat Recipe 80 percent]

Fresco Fried Queso [1/3 Lb Fried Queso]

841 Calories, 57.3 g Fats, 0.2 g Net Carbs, and 75.2 g Protein per serving.

Dessert

[Eat 1 Spice Cake] Low Carb Spice Cake

283 Calories, 27 g Fats, 3.3 g Net Carbs, and 7.3 g Protein per serving.

Totals for the day

1670 Calories, 144.3 g of fat, 5 g of net Carbs and 82.5 g of protein

Day 21

Breakfast

Bulletproof [Double serving] Coffee

546 Calories, 60 g Fats, 1.5 g Net Carbs, and 0 g Protein per serving.

Lunch

Fast through lunch, make sure you have plenty of water to drink!

Dinner

Left Bacon Explosion [Eat 1 serving] [Use Leftovers] [Add 4 Spinach Cups]

748 Calories, 63.7 g Fats, 5.9 g Net Carbs, and 57.7 g Protein per serving.

Dessert

[Eat 1 Spice Cake] Low Carb Spice Cake

283 Calories, 27 g Fats, 3.3 g Net Carbs, and 7.3 g Protein per serving.

Totals for the day

1577 Calories, 150.7 g of fats, 10.7 g of net Carbs and 65 g of protein

Week 4

We're becoming more intense with our fasting this week. We have had a full week of intermittent fasting, and we will now skip breakfast and lunch. Our BEST friend here is Water! Don't forget to drink coffee, tea, flavored water, and put in your beverages. Keep on drinking to make sure you don't care about your stomach. It MIGHT begin growling, just ignore it- with time your body can change.

If you're the kind of person who can't fast, you can go back and follow up again on week 2. That's not such a big deal. It takes the body some time to fast, though, so I suggest putting your best efforts into it. The health benefits good, but it's also cool to have the self-control you achieve from doing so.

This is my favorite week with a great deal because it most closely resembles how I eat every day. I usually set a 6-hour window for me to eat in. I fast from waking up till 5 pm. Afterward, I'm available until 11 pm to eat. This is where the fun begins. Eat lots of food and be full to the next day. You get to begin more dessert and dinner experiments. You get to snack inside your window as you like and the best of all – you get to eat the protein-laden chicken you've missed so much!

Breakfast.

We are on the quick! Black coffee, if you are an addict of caffeine like me. Tea, if you're not that much into the coffee. Unlike coffee, tea will have significant health benefits too. Several of the great benefits of green tea are Polyphenols – These function in your body as antioxidants. Epigallocatechin gallate (EGCG) is the most potent antioxidant in green tea, protective against fatigue.

Better brain activity – Green tea not only includes caffeine but also contains L-theanine, an amino acid. L-theanine increases GABA production, thus boosting waves of fear, dopamine, and alpha. Increased metabolic rate-It has been shown that green tea can increase the metabolic rate. Along with the caffeine, this can lead to fat oxidation of up to 15 percent.

Lunch.

Water and Water, and then a little more Water. You can't eat lunch, and you can't eat brunch. So make sure you remain hydrated ALWAY. Whether you do a decent job with your hydration is imperative here. Recall-I suggests 4 liters a day.

Dinner.

Lots and lots of dessert food to cover the bases! Dinner is a wonderful time for me. I recommend you break your fast with a small snack, then eat to your heart's content after 30-45 minutes. I usually need 2 meals to get to my macros, and I guess you'll have to do the same thing.

Shopping List for Week 4

Meat

Ground Chicken

Fats

Sesame Oil

Sauces

1 Can Coors Light

Chili Garlic Paste

Reduced Sugar Ketchup

Crunch

Peanuts (or peanut butter)

Pumpkin Seeds

Cheese

Blue Cheese Crumbles

Cream Cheese

Mozzarella Cheese

Spices

CapersFive-Spice

Red Food Coloring

Day 22

Breakfast

We fast for breakfast. With no ingredients added, you can drink black coffee or tea. You should also drink water during breakfast. I strongly suggest drinking plenty of water.

Lunch

We fast for lunch. With no ingredients added, you can drink black coffee or tea. Try not to go beyond three cups of coffee or tea a day, though. You can also drink water-through lunch. I highly recommend drinking plenty of water.

Dinner

Keto Style Szechuan Chicken [Freeze Leftoversas 2 Portions] [Eat 1/3 Total Recipe]

Pecan Roasted Green Beans [Eat 1 serving] [Use Leftovers]

697 Calories, 55.2 g Fats, 8.5 g Net Carbs, and 66.7 g Protein per serving.

Dessert

Cakes in Almond Lemon Sandwich [Eat 4 Sandwich Cakes]

[Write 1 Tbsp. Butter [butter]

819 Calories, 81 g Fats, 7.3 g Net Carbs, and 11.2 g Protein per serving.

Totals for the day

1517 Calories, Fats 136.2 g, Net Carbs 15.9 g, and Protein 77.9g

Day 23

Breakfast

We fast for breakfast. With no ingredients added, you can drink black coffee or tea. You should also drink water during breakfast. I strongly suggest drinking plenty of water.

Lunch

We fast for lunch. With no ingredients added, you can drink black coffee or tea. Try not to go beyond three cups of coffee or tea a day, though. You can also drink water-through lunch. I highly recommend drinking plenty of water.

Dinner

Leftover Meatballs [Eat 5 Meatballs] [Eat 5 Meatballs]

Cheesy Creamed Spinach [Freeze Leftovers] [Eat 1/2 of Recipe]

1061 Calories, 93.1 g Fats, 8.5 g Net Carbs, 60.6 g Protein per serving.

Dessert

Chai Spice Cake for Mug [Add 2 Tbsp. Crème Heavy]

539 Calories, 52 g Fats, 5.2 g Net Carbs, and 12 g Protein per serving.

Day Total

S1600 Calories, 145,1 g of fats, 13,7 g of net Carbs and 72,6 g of protein

Day 24

Breakfast

We fast for breakfast. With no ingredients added, you can drink black coffee or tea. You should also drink water during breakfast. I strongly suggest drinking plenty of water.

Lunch

We fast for lunch. With no ingredients added, you can drink black coffee or tea. Try not to go beyond three cups of coffee or tea a day, though. You can also drink water-through lunch. I highly recommend drinking plenty of water.

Dinner

Curry Rubbed Thigh Chicken [Make 3 Thigh Chicken]

Vegetable Medley [Freeze Leftovers] [Eat 1/3 of Recipe]

1069 Calories, 83.7 g Fats, 9.3 g Net Carbs, and 63 g Protein per serving.

Dessert

Cakes in Almond Lemon Sandwich [Eat 3 Sandwich Cakes]

539 Calories, 52.5 g Fats, 5.5 g Net Carbs, and 8.4 g Protein per serving.

Complete day

S1609 Calories, 136.2 g Fat, 14.8 g Net Carb, and 71.4 g Protein

Day 25

Breakfast

We fast for breakfast. With no ingredients added, you can drink black coffee or tea. You should also drink water during breakfast. I strongly suggest drinking plenty of water.

Lunch

We fast for lunch. With no ingredients added, you can drink black coffee or tea. Try not to go beyond three cups of coffee or tea a day, though. You can also drink water-through lunch. I highly recommend drinking plenty of water.

Dinner

Thai Style Peanut Chicken [Freeze Leftovers] [Eat 1/2 of Recipe]

Easy [2 Cups Spinach salad, 2 Tbsp. Palm oil: Olive oil]

1003 Calories, 81.5 g Fats, 9.3 g Net Carbs, and 72 g Protein per serving.

Dessert

Cakes in Almond Lemon Sandwich [Eat 3 Sandwich Cakes]

539 Calories, 52.5 g Fats, 5.5 g Net Carbs, and 8.4 g Protein per serving.

Complete day

S1543 Calories, 134 g Fat, 14.7 g Net Carbs, and 80.4 g Protein

Day 26

Breakfast

We fast for breakfast. With no ingredients added, you can drink black coffee or tea. You should also drink water during breakfast. I strongly suggest drinking plenty of water.

Lunch

We fast for lunch. With no ingredients added, you can drink black coffee or tea. Try not to go beyond three cups of coffee or tea a day, though. You can also drink water-through lunch. I highly recommend drinking plenty of water.

Dinner

Coffee & Wine Beef Stew [Freeze Leftovers as 3 Portions] [Eat 1/4 of Recipe]

Spinach salad [2 Spinach tassels, 2 Tbsp. Palm oil: Olive oil]

1015 Calories, 76.3 g Fats, 4.5 g Net Carbs, and 65.3 g Protein per serving.

Dessert

Chai Spice Cake for Mug [Add 3 Tbsp. Crème Heavy]

589 Calories, 57 g Fats, 5.8 g Net Carbs, and 12 g Protein per serving.

Complete day

S1605 Calories, Fats 133.3 g, Net Carbs 10.3 g, and Protein 77.3g

Day 27

Breakfast

We fast for breakfast. With no ingredients added, you can drink black coffee or tea. You should also drink water during breakfast. I strongly suggest drinking plenty of water.

Lunch

We fast for lunch. With no ingredients added, you can drink black coffee or tea. Try not to go beyond three cups of coffee or tea a day, though. You can also drink water-through lunch. I highly recommend drinking plenty of water.

Dinner

Drunken Five-Spice Beef [Freeze Leftovers] [Eating 1/2 of Recipe]

1030 Calories, 70 g Fats, 12 g Net Carbs, and 66.5 g Protein per serving

Dessert

Cookies with Keto Snickerdoodle [Eat 4 Cookies]

528 Calories, 49.6 g Fats, 8 g Net Carbs and 13.7 g Protein per serving

Totals for the day

1558 Calories, Fats 119.6 g, Net Carbs 20 g, and Protein 80.2 g

Day 28

Breakfast

We fast for breakfast. With no ingredients added, you can drink black coffee or tea. You should also drink water during breakfast. I strongly suggest drinking plenty of water.

Lunch

We fast for lunch. With no ingredients added, you can drink black coffee or tea. Try not to go beyond three cups of coffee or tea a day, though. You can also drink water-through lunch. I highly recommend drinking plenty of water.

Dinner

Lemon & Rosemary Roasted Thighs for Chicken [Eat the Whole Recipe]

Red Spinach Pepper Salad [Eat 1/2 Recipe]

797 Calories, 58.5 g Fats, 7.7 g Net Carbs, and 55 g Protein per serving.

Dessert

Cookies Keto Snickerdoodle [Eat 6 Cookies]

792 Calories, 74.4 g Fats, 12 g Net Carbs, and 20.6 g Protein per serving.

Complete day

S1589 Calories, 132.9 g Fat, 19.7 g Net Carbs, and 75.6 g Protein